Thank You

Before we begin I would like to thank Jonathon, the Mac geek, for coming up with this title and sharing that some people don't want to study a big book, that many people just want the facts, the tips and instructions on how they can be better, feel better and get back to their vibrant life.

I was inspired as soon as I heard the title and saw the graphic that he created.

Thank you! Thank you!

An Ounce of Prevention
Help Everyday Ailments Naturally

"I have learned so much from Sheila's books and teachings. What she does really works. I even did her full 8 weeks to Wellness program. "I cannot say enough about how my life and my business has soared. I never knew success could feel so good and I can say with 100% certainty that getting my health back is the foundation of this amazing life. I am so grateful for all the research, and education and even yummy meals that made such an amazing difference. Myself and my entire family are so grateful."

Karen

"I have know Sheila for many years. She has changed my health for the better, her books and CD's have been an inspiration. I also went through her 8 week program that was amazing. "The program was an incredible journey that was really like going to a private college. Including a wide array of subjects all pertaining to my own health and wellness. It changed my life and my health for the better in a huge way. And now I have everything I need to stay well for the next 100 years. It seems that my health issues in many areas were all resolved.
From the bottom of my heart, Thank you"

Cheri

"I have followed Sheila's work for many years.
I had so many ailments including a diagnosis of pending cancer. I actually took an extended 3 month program, it saved my life. "When I started My numbers were a mess. I had many ailments and had just been diagnosed with pending prostate cancer on top of high sugar. I knew I had to do something and immediately. After being on the program my life changed. My numbers came back into normal range, all of my numbers. It was like a miracle and I can honestly say this saved my life"

Steve G.

The Healer Within
The concept of the healer within is not new, only forgotten.
"Natural forces within us are the true healers of disease."
Spoken and written by Hippocrates (460 – 357 BC)

Let's think about the above statement for a moment.

This means that 460 years before the birth of Christ, people knew they were the driving force in their own healing and wellness. So, what happened? Through the ages there have been healers, those who heard the call, in tribes and clans. There were men and women who knew every plant and every stone—and the healthful uses for these great tools for healing.

It may be that the time has come to look back on some of these natural ways and ideas. A time to know how amazing our bodies are if we can just give our bodies the correct tools to work with. And there is where the idea and practice of prevention will thrive once again.

Benjamin Franklin - made this original quote.
The Benjamin Franklin axiom that;
    "An ounce of prevention is worth a pound of cure"
is as true today as it was when Ben Franklin made the quote. Although many use the quote when referring to health, Franklin was actually addressing fire safety. Franklin wrote this under an assumed name.
(courtesy of ushistory.org)

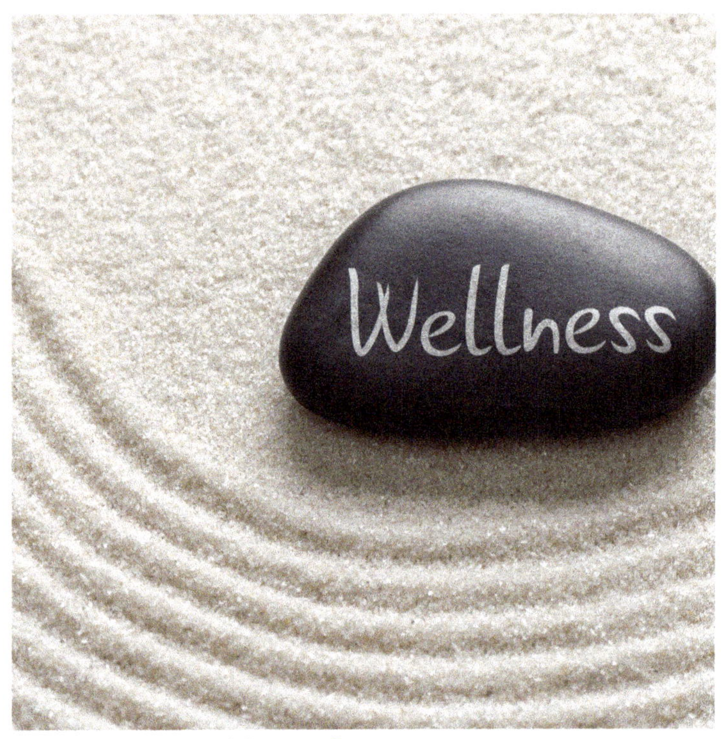

About Prevention

Let's talk about prevention and why you would want get on board with this train of thought.

Regardless if you are 20 or 90 years young, we all know many people who are suffering from so many different small ailments and maybe some are suffering from some large ailments.

Let's start with the true statement that *"The body wants to be well."* This is one of many quotes of mine and I know this is **100% true!** At some point,

I think I say that to everyone who crosses my path. *Because, it is the truth!* You have around 100 trillion cells in your body and each one is a miracle unto itself.

Think about it for a moment...
even the act of breathing is a miracle!

We breathe in oxygen from the air, and in an instant every cell takes in oxygen and exhales the carbon dioxide which is the by-product, the exhaust system that allows us to take the next breath.

If we did not have a vibrant plant life on this planet, this exchange would be in real trouble. The trees, and the plant life breathe in the carbon dioxide and expel oxygen which we then breath in... etc... etc… it is a symbiotic relationship between the human world and the plant world. A delicate balance to be sure.

Life is meant to be a wiggle not a struggle.
(Sheila Z)

So, where do we start on this journey of preventing dis-ease and age related challenges?

Let's start at a place I believe we all want to be. That is...to **be better, feel better, do better** and yes, even **look better!** And, to avoid the challenges our parents had as they matured. To stay young and vibrant regardless of your age or your family's history.

In many countries "prevention" is revered, and thought of as the best way to approach your health and wellness. Unfortunately, in the United States it is not exactly easy, as most all allopathic doctors were not really trained in prevention. Don't get me wrong, I admire and honor the allopathic physician that goes through the ten to fourteen years of schooling and opens a practice–*"practice"* being the operative word. Our doctors are great at handing out pills and great advise in many cases. And, you definitely want an allopathic to be performing surgery if the time comes when you may need that sort of treatment.

Prevention starts early and takes education. For it is true; knowledge is power. Preventing some age related illnesses is a cornerstone of a long happy and vibrant life.
Here are just a few examples of conditions we can prevent all together or lesson the impact. In almost all cases we can knock down many symptoms that impact the quality of your life, or the life of a loved one. Please remember, this is *my* opinion.

• Diabetes	• IBS
• Metabolic Syndrome	• Crone's Disease
• Heart Disease	• MS
• Kidney Disease	• Mental Fog
• Breathing Challenges	• Depression
• Digestive Challenges	• Fatigue
• Memory Loss	• Obesity

Along with all the newly named disorders like Fibromyalgia, Chronic Fatigue and so much more. Regardless of what is happening, realize that gaining the right and true tools on health and wellness can change everything for the better.

An Ounce of Prevention is more of a guide. In it you will find specific tips and facts to help your everyday life to be more vibrant, more alive and yes, there will be overlaps about using food as medicine. As repetition is how we learn so dive right in and enjoy.

A thought on Prevention: One day you look out and it's cloudy outside. You are all dressed up for a meeting and know you do NOT want to get wet. So, you bring a hat and an umbrella with you so your day will go smoothly and you will stay dry.

Prevention is just like that. You look out on your life and think "I want to feel great and be happy regardless of my age or the season." So, you educate yourself in the ways of being and staying healthy to avoid the "pit falls" of aging.

Prevention is your umbrella in life. So welcome, step right in and set yourself free.

The 4 Pillars of Health & Wellness

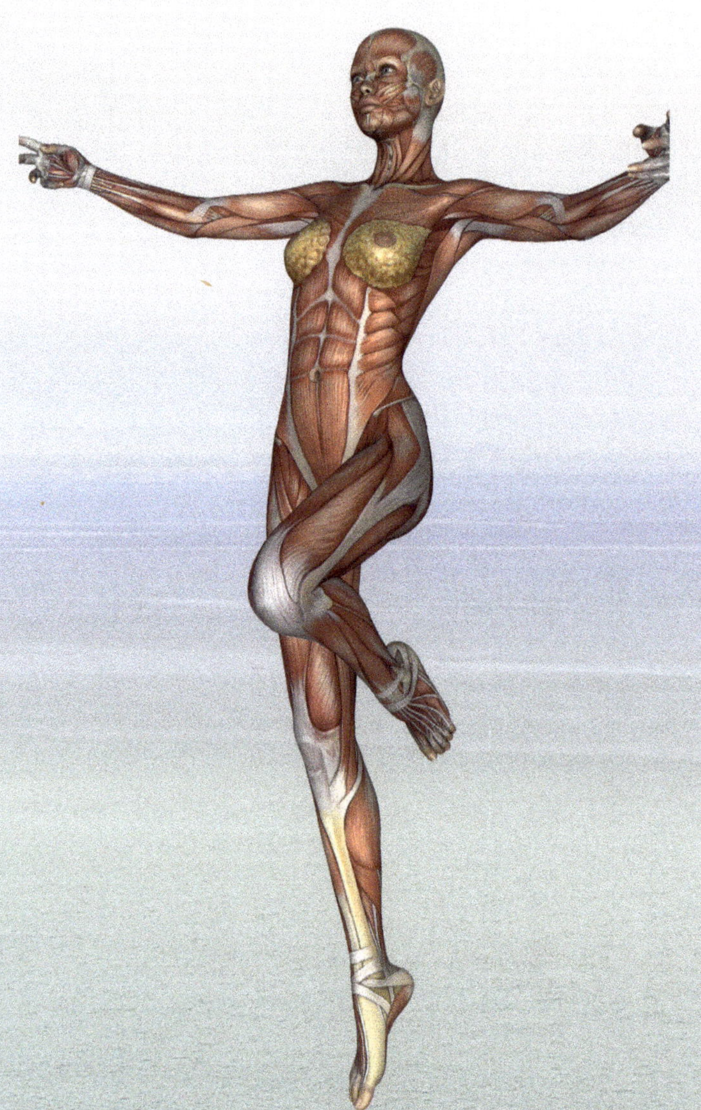

4 Pillars of Wellness

In my big book *"Anatomy of Healing and Wellness"* I discuss what I call the *4 Pillars of Health and Wellness*. I dive into the organs, the physical body, the science of wellness and the emotional aspect of health and wellness. And, the last chapters are focused on *Using Food as Medicine,* including herbs, teas and spices. In this writing the 4 pillars may seem to be all mixed in and I assure you, I cover them all.

I promise to keep this reference under 180 pages where *Anatomy of Healing and Wellness* book is over 268 pages in an oversized format. Although, there are some excerpts from the *Anatomy of Healing and Wellness* in this guide, it is all great cutting-edge information.

The time has come to realize that Allopathic physicians were not trained to really assist you in regaining your wellness. They might have had a day or two of instruction on nutrition, but when it comes to the chemistry of what food does once it is digested, it would be a foreign language for most. So, we must now realize that it is time to take control of our own well being and take responsibility and the steps it takes to keep (or reclaim) our vibrant health and wellness.

As we age, some things become more important:
- Like understanding our digestive system, understanding how to keep our bodies limber and working on all 1,000 cylinders.

- Like knowing that 70% of your lymphatic system resides in your gut!

- Knowing that your pancreas actually takes some instruction from your liver.

- Knowing that certain levels need to be maintained in the body in order to "stay 30 until you are 90." This is the motto of my company and also how I speak to every cell in my body every day.

- Knowing that your belief system effects every cell in your body.

- Knowing that NOW is the perfect time to embrace your amazing wellness.

So, let's go through the
4 Pillars of Health & Wellness
and learn how to keep young, beautiful
and inspired everyday of your life.

First, let us enter the realm of the Physical Form

Below are some facts everyone needs to know: This chapter talks of breath and your vital organs, so read on.

#1: Let's talk about breath & breathing.

I know I brought it up in the beginning and now let's dive a bit deeper. This includes blood pressure, heart rate and a few foods that are heart friendly.

Your entire body is made up of thousands of different pathways—that all interact and share connections and information. They work together in a symbiotic relationship. Take breathing for example. Just breathe in… now let's take a look at what just happened. As you breathe in, the cilia (tiny hairs) in the nose begin to filter out particles, the cells are alerted of the incoming oxygen, and every cell responds as the lungs fill. The bloodstream absorbs oxygen and the brain is revitalized with the incoming life giving element of air. And then, as miraculous as it came in, we exhale and expel the carbon dioxide our bodies cannot use or assimilate.

However, the plant life on this planet lives and thrives on this carbon dioxide and takes it in, turns it back into oxygen and expels it … and we breathe it in. How's that for a symbiotic relationship? A very good reason to be sure that the plant kingdom on this planet is happy and thriving. For we are directly connected to their well-being.

Yes, the miles of veins, arteries, and 100 trillion cells, are all reborn with every breath we take in. It seems like an impossible mission, and it is all put together without us having to consciously think about it. When we breathe out or exhale, all the used molecules are drawn from the cells, organs, muscles and tissue, and expelled into the atmosphere. Then the cycle begins again.

3 Stages of Breath
(This is my concept of course)

There are 3 stages of breathing.

Have you ever watched a baby breathe? This is **Stage 1** breathing. The deep breath of an infant seems to come from their stomach (belly). It rises as their lungs fill with air. And then, contracts as they exhale.

Now think about how most people breathe.

Stage 2 breath seems to come from the diaphragm (we hope). The air expands the lungs and each breath renews you. There is no rising and falling of the shoulders at all. The lungs expand outwards from all sides. If your shoulders are moving...you are not getting the oxygen you need. Most people are breathing somewhere between stages 2 and 3.

Now, take a look at someone close to crossing over or transitioning. This is **Stage 3** of breathing. They breathe from their upper chest and throat, moving their shoulders (or maybe not) with every breath. And, in the final stage of stage 3 the breath becomes very shallow, almost like a gasp as the last breath is expelled for the final time.
This should occur when you're over 125 years of age. Yes, that is correct. With our bodies and cells constantly renewing themselves, why do some people age so quickly?

Regardless of where you are or your chronological age, start breathing in a way that oxygenates your body. It may add many happy healthier years to your life.

Stage 1 breathing is a must if you want to stay 30 till you are 90. *Here is how to practice:*

Lay on the floor if you can and place a good sized book on your belly. You may also lay on a bed or flat surface if laying on the floor is difficult for you.

Now, breathe in through your nose, filling your lungs as they expand outward. Watch the book as it should also move up and down with each breath. Notice where your shoulders are and make sure they are not moving. Practice makes perfect, so go ahead and try it. It's also a good test to be sure you are breathing in a way that will enhance your life. Remember, your lungs fill like billows, expanding like a balloon.

Let's talk about

#2 Blood Pressure

since it is related to breathing.
Oh, yes it is!

How many people over 40 are on blood pressure medication? Really the number is staggering.

How many deaths are related or caused by high blood pressure? **Here is what Google says:** *"Blood pressure in the United States is a primary or contributing cause of death is about 350,000 in a year. That is almost 1,000 deaths each day. 7 of every 10 people having their first heart attack have high blood pressure."*

Did you know there are many natural alternatives to medication and many natural ways to bring your blood pressure down?

1. A good cardiologist will tell you about a device called **"Resperate."** It basically teaches you how to breathe in order to bring your pressure

into normal range. You strap it around your upper ribs and it learns your rhythm and tells you when to inhale and when to exhale. It trains you to breathe correctly.

2. The Breath of Life (as I call it). You breathe in through your nose and from your belly. This should be about 2-4 seconds and then exhale through your lips that are narrowed (like you're blowing out your birthday candles). This needs to take about 8-10 seconds. This breathing will also train your brain and have your blood pressure normalizing. You can do this when you are taking a walk or sitting quietly.

3. Magnesium Malate: This form of magnesium relaxes your arteries and naturally causes your blood pressure to come down. You can buy this at any health food store. Just be sure it is "Malate." You can just chew a half or whole one and then drink some water. If you take too much it can give you loose stools. This is a good fact to know.

4. Really warm/very warm water will also relax your entire vascular system. Soaking your feet up to your ankles has proven to be very effective as well.

5. *How about slowing down a fast heart rate?* Yes, you can! And please note that sometimes a fast heart rate actually means your blood pressure may be low and your heart has to pump extra hard to keep the blood oxygen flowing. You will

need to inhale through your nose, blocking one nostril, then exhale through your nose blocking the other nostril so only one nostril is blocked at a time. Sit down and do this for about 5 minutes and you will feel you heart beat regulating.

Before we move on, I would like to share with you the importance of *"pulse pressure."* In my opinion, this is the most important number of the blood pressure reading. *What the heck is that?* you may ask...since your doctor never really told you about it. Well, it is the most important number because it lets you know the percentage of the pressure against your arteries. So, 120/80 has a pulse pressure of 40 – a perfect place to be keeping your "PP" (Pulse Pressure) in the range of 40-50 is ideal.

Let's say you have low blood pressure like 114/70, your pulse pressure would be 44 that is actually really good. What if your pressure is 117/64 your pp would be 53 still not too bad. What if it is 145/85 your pp would be 60...not so great! Getting the picture? You subtract the bottom number from the top and there you have it.

How about 117/41 your pulse pressure would be 76 so even though your pressure is low the pulse pressure can be high. In this case, you want to watch that your pulse number is not high and around the 60 or 70 range. If it is very high like 90 or above or very low like 40 or below you may want to visit your friendly cardiologist.

I hope these few tips have been useful for your everyday life. They don't call high blood pressure the silent killer for nothing. The fact is if you have not treated your high blood pressure you are running a risky game–as your arteries and capillaries are like rubber bands and what happens to a rubber band that is constantly being stretched out? Yes, it becomes weak and more apt to break.

So, take care of your blood pressure and it will take good care of you.

I would like to add that having a blood pressure cuff at home in never a bad idea.

You can get them on amazon and they are not expensive. Ask your doctor which kind he recommends. Same with a oxygen meter. It is small and not expensive and takes only a minute or so to see where your oxygen levels are at.

Let's move on to some Tips on Your Organs

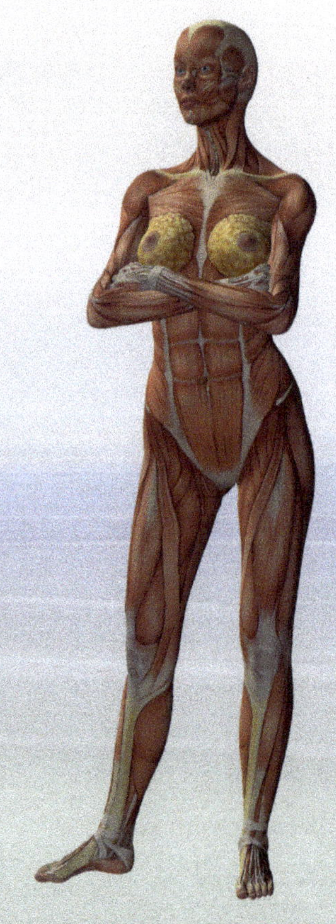

Why you ask? Because, in today's world where the minerals are depleted in the soil and the water is fluorinated (which is a poison) and the air is full of particalized barium, strontium and aluminum, it's a wonder any of us are living at all.

Now, we must take responsibility for the level of health and wellness we desire. You can make it happen or you can allow it to fall by the wayside. Ultimately, the choice is yours.

Some time ago a friend was telling me how difficult his life was. He was in a relationship that was NOT in his best interest and he was making poor choices when it came to food and into gaining the truthful knowledge that would change his life for the better. I told him, "It is your choice." You can choose to live a healthy happy life and surround yourself with truly caring people or you can choose to do nothing and simply go on until that day comes when your body, mind and spirit says "no more." You must choose to LIVE OR DIE. I am not kidding about that. It really comes down to that simple question. So, I ask you now...what is your answer?

If your choice is to live then please read on.

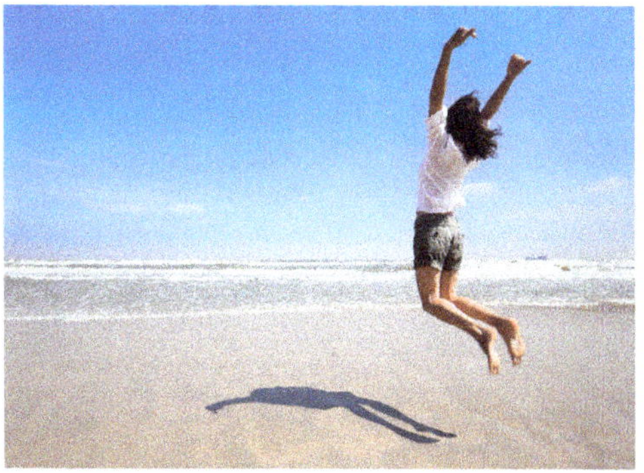

The Liver

Let's talk about what I call your master organ, (or, at least one of them). Yes, most people look at the heart as the master but for today's purpose we are referring to the liver. This amazing organ not only detoxifies the body, it also processes nutrients from food, makes bile, removes toxins from the body, and builds proteins. In fact, the liver's main function is to filter the blood coming from the digestive tract before passing it to the rest of the body.

It's easy to see how inflammation, (or hepatitis) of the liver, fatty liver interferes with these important functions and can lead to poor health. You do not have to have hepatitis for your liver to get bogged down and clogged. It's a good thing the liver is so resilient, and will usually respond to herbs, foods and a number of natural methods that will keep your liver happy. And a happy liver means a happy you!

Here are a few tips that can help you help your liver to keep you young and strong:

1. Eat lots of Organic Arugula!
It is considered a bitter and bitters help improve the bile production in the liver. This in turn improves your overall health.

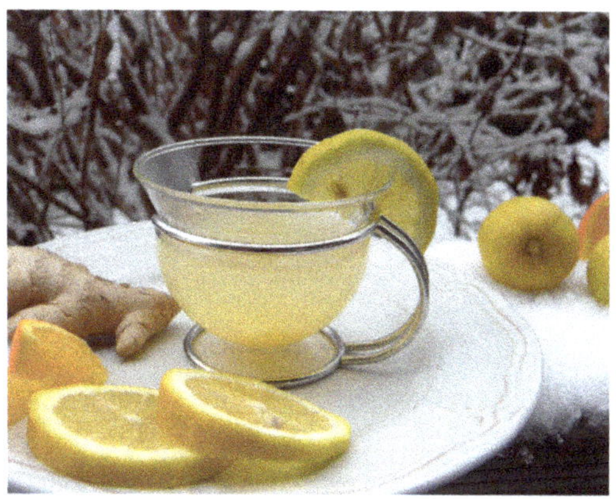

2. Lemon Water first thing in the morning is a great way to start your day. It's amazing what just a squeeze of "organic lemon" can do for your health and wellness.

(excerpt from Anatomy of Healing and Wellness)

Lemon is an excellent, rich source of Vitamin C, an essential nutrient that protects the body against immune system deficiencies.

Lemons contain pectin fiber, which is very beneficial for colon health, and also serves as a powerful antibacterial.

- It balances and maintains the pH levels in the body.

- It is an acid that turns alkaline in the body. If you are at 7.0 - 7.2 pH—all is great. Most people are lower than this, and as our bodies fall to a lower pH—there are many diseases that may find it easier to take hold.

- Having warm lemon water early in the morning helps flush out toxins.

- It has a synergizing effect on the body, as it helps soothe the digestive system.

- It aids digestion and encourages the production of bile.

- It conditions and helps cleanses the liver.

- It is also a great source of citric acid, potassium, calcium, phosphorus and magnesium.

- It helps prevent the growth and multiplication of pathogenic bacteria that cause infections and diseases.

Here are a few more benefits of lemons:
- They help maintain the health of the eyes and help to fight against eye problems.

- Lemons aid in the reduction of phlegm (mucus) produced by the body.

- Lemon helps control the spreading of unhealthy bacteria in the gut.

- Lemons aid in the production of digestive juices. The warm water serves to stimulate the gastrointestinal tract and peristalsis—the waves of muscle contractions within the intestinal walls that keep things moving. Lemons and limes are also high in minerals and Vitamins which help loosen toxins, in the digestive tract.

- Lemons can treat a sore throat. Gargle with warm lemon water to help ease a sore throat.

Adopting, just this one practice of drinking a cup of warm water with lemon in the morning for a month, can radically alter your experience of the day. Don't be surprised if you begin to view mornings in a new light. Remember, much of the phyto-nutrients are in the peel so don't be shy, put a little bit of peel in there as well.

Stay hydrated with water. Soft drinks just gum up your organs.

3. Milk Thistle

The herb Milk Thistle is good for protecting your liver and can be bought as a loose herb. just half a teaspoon is great mixed in a smoothie or sprinkled over a salad.

Milk Thistle is one of the many herbs that has been used for 2,000 years in many herbal remedies for a variety of ailments, particularly liver, kidney, and gall bladder problems. Several scientific studies suggest that substances in Milk Thistle protect the liver from toxins, including certain drugs such as acetaminophen (Tylenol), which can cause liver damage in high doses. Milk Thistle (Silymarin) has antioxidant and anti-inflammatory properties, and it may help the liver repair itself by growing new cells. Here again, anti-oxidation is key in revitalizing the liver. *From my Anatomy of Healing and Wellness book*

Also certain foods are a great way to keep your liver healthy. They include:
- Garlic
- Beets
- Grapefruit
- Green Tea
- Leafy Green Veggies
- Avocados
- Green Apples
- Organic Olive Oil
- And of course Lemons and Limes

...just to name a few. *(I go into depth on this in my "Anatomy of Healing and Wellness Book")*

Your Beautiful Heart

According to U.S. Health Statistics:
Cardiovascular disease claims more lives each year than any major diagnostic group. Coronary heart disease accounted for approximately 13% of deaths in the U.S. Someone has a stroke every 40 seconds on average–killing approximately 142,000 people a year.

A Better Heart: As identified by Arab L. (et al.) in their 2009 research paper called *"Green and Black Tea Consumption and Risk of Stroke: a Meta-analysis"*–it is seen that regardless of people's country of origin, individuals who consume 3 or more cups of tea had a 21% lower risk of a stroke than people who consume less than 1 cup of green or black tea per day. It seems like such an easy task and yet, how many cups of tea are you drinking every day?

Here are a few tips to help out.

Tip 1: The Cleveland Clinic agrees (as do so many other research papers and institutions) that simply by brushing and flossing your teeth every day actually assists in keeping your heart healthy. Here is a little known fact as well; men are more susceptible to heart related illnesses due to the health of their teeth than women.

Still, we all need to be aware of the direct correlation between the health of our mouth and our hearts. In fact, gum disease can move into the bloodstream and cause an elevation in C-reactive protein, a marker for inflammation in the blood vessels and that in turn can up your risk of a cardiovascular event. A simple blood test called CRP will measure your inflammation level. This is a very good number to know.

Tip 2: Remember, your heart is a muscle, an amazing multifaceted muscle. Keeping active is a cornerstone for keeping all our muscles in good condition and that includes your heart. So, get up off your chair and walk, dance, box, skate, hike or do what ever makes you happy in the way of movement. And remember, sex is also very good for your heart in so many ways.

Tip 3: Yes! do eat heart healthy foods and that includes healthy fats! Like avocado, coconut oil, pure olive oil. Look for 0% trans fats as they are terrible for your heart. I believe in the "Using food as Medicine" ideal and in that section there are many more on the list.

Your Kidneys

Google says it so simply: "The kidneys are two bean-shaped organs in the renal system. They help the body pass waste as urine. They also help filter blood before sending it back to the heart. Yes, your kidneys are an amazing purification mechanism, by filtering your blood of impurities."

There are many foods that can assist to keep your kidneys strong. Below are eight foods that are great tips on how to feed good nutrition to your kidneys.

Tip 1: *Eat foods that are healthy for your kidneys:*
1. Cabbage (½ cup serving green cabbage = 6 mg sodium, 60 mg potassium, 9 mg phosphorus)
2. Cauliflower
3. Garlic
4. Onions
5. Apples.
6. Dark Leafy Greens
7. Cranberries
8. Blueberries

Tip 2: Drink plenty of water! Just water! Remember, soft drinks or sugary drinks are not good for your kidneys or any other part of your body.

Tip 3: Yes, keeping fit is a good thing. Also, if you smoke...STOP! Stop now!

Tip 4: Maintain a healthy weight as everything effects your kidneys. They are a major filtration system and an unsung hero of your wellness goals.

Tip 5: Please note that your blood sugar and blood pressure also have an effect on your kidneys. Make sure your numbers are in a good place and if they are not...change it now as you really do not want to mess with kidney problems. Your kidneys have many more functions and it may be a good idea to know them.

Did you know kidneys assist in:
- Maintaining your Electrolyte balance.
- Assists in controlling blood pressure and water balance in your body.
- Controls the acid-base balance in your body.
- Produces the hormone Erythropoietin which stimulates bone marrow and helps develop red blood cells.
- The kidneys also activate Vitamin D.

So let's keep our kidneys very happy...ok?

Your Colon

The colon is part of the large intestine, the final part of the digestive system. Its function is to re-absorb fluids and process waste products from the body and prepare for its elimination. The colon consists of four parts: descending colon, ascending colon, transverse colon, and sigmoid colon.

Eating high fiber foods like fresh organic berries and organic fruits and vegetables are great for your colon. Eating processed meats and processed foods are the opposite.

IBS
(Irritable Bowel Syndrome)

Irritable Bowel Syndrome (IBS). This can be caused by many things or a combinations of things and really is the increased sensitivity of the nerves in your digestive tract.

Tip 1: As a digestive; **cinnamon** dramatically reduces the uncomfortable feelings associated with IBS—especially the bloating. It does this by killing bacteria and healing infections in the GI tract and enabling the gastric juices to work normally. A Japanese study showed it to cure ulcers, but this cannot be verified. But, if you do have stomach cramps or upsets, **a cup of Cinnamon tea 2-3 times per day will dramatically reduce the pain.**

Tip 2: Drinking warm water or a nice hot cup of tea may relax your muscles. Even using a hot water bottle may help.

Tip 3: Magnesium (or a product named **CALM**) may assist if you are also constipated. This can make everything feel better as waste is toxic to the body and can cause you to feel really bad.

Diverticulosis and Diverticulitis
are called diverticular disease.

Google says it well: "Diverticulitis most commonly affects the sigmoid colon, which is the last part of the large intestine just before the rectum."

Diverticular disease can develop in any part of the digestive tract, but it affects the large intestine, or colon, most often. Diverticulitis is an infected pouch in the colon. Symptoms of diverticulitis include pain, constipation, and blood in the stool.

One of the main causes of diverticular disease is thought to be a lack of dietary fiber.

*There are many food that will **NOT** flare up this condition here are just a few:*
- White rice, white bread, or white pasta, but avoid gluten-containing foods if you're intolerant.

- Dry, low-fiber cereals.

- Processed fruits such as applesauce or canned peaches.

- Cooked animal proteins such as fish, poultry, or eggs.

- Olive oil or other oils.

- Basically very low fiber foods.

There are also many foods you should NOT eat!
- Certain fruits, like apples, pears, and plums.
- Dairy foods, such as milk, yogurt, ice cream.
- Fermented foods, such as sauerkraut or kimchi.
- Beans and Cabbage.
- Brussels sprouts.
- Onions and garlic.
- The skin on veggies and fruits.

What about nuts you ask?
In the past, doctors recommended that people with diverticulitis avoid eating nuts, popcorn, and most seeds. It was thought that the tiny particles from these foods might get lodged in the pouches and lead to an infection. As a rule walnuts may be ok if you chew them to a liquid. Small seeds and most nuts may trigger an attack.

*So, now we have covered many organs,
let's turn our attention to some
everyday situations...*

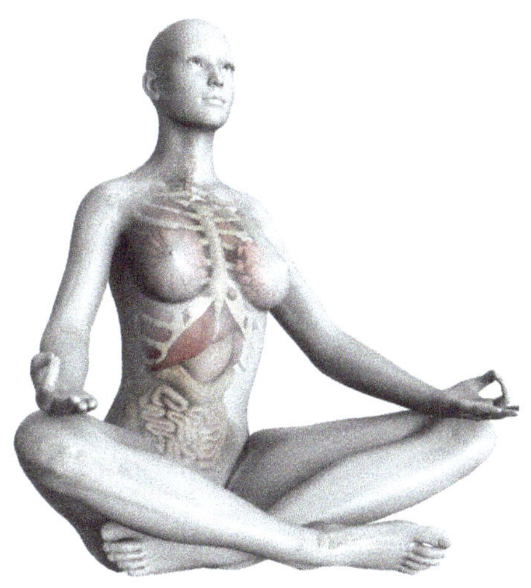

How To Prevent a Cold:

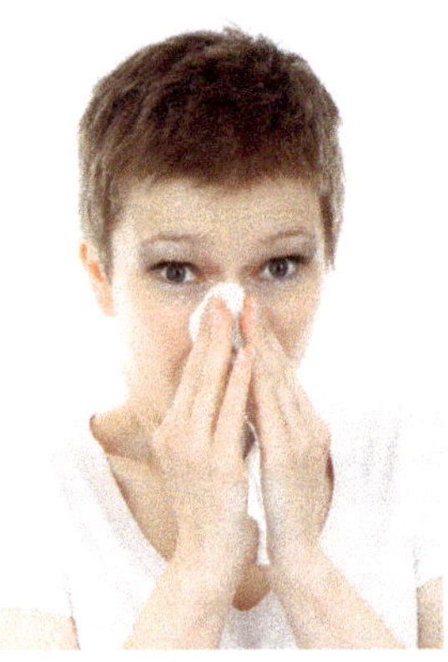

Tip 1: Stop shaking hands! 97% of viruses are passed through the palm of the hand. Wash your hands often and do not touch your eyes, nose or mouth.

Tip 2: Cover your ears when there is wind or cold. You need to realize that many viruses are airborne and are carried on the breeze. Your ears are an opening...we seem to forget about that.

Tip 3: Be sure your Vitamin D3 levels are good as well as Vitamin C and remember, absorbic acid is NOT Vitamin C, your liver has to convert it. The truth is Vitamin D3 is actually a hormone and not a vitamin at all. It is great for your immune system, bones, brain and so much more. Get tested and make sure your levels are good and supplement if you are a bit low.

What About Viruses?

Today, that seems to be at the forefront of everyone's concern. So, let's take the mystery out of this situation. First of all, the best way to keep from getting a virus is to keep your immune system strong. Your body was meant to not only fight a virus, but it also has the ability to build the antibody it needs, so you will more than likely not get the same strain again.

The Top 3 Tips are:

Tip 1: Keep your hands and face really clean. Wash with soap! Keep washing your hands for 20 seconds or more.

Tip 2: Boost your citrus intake, such as organic grapefruit, lemons, oranges and kiwi. These fruits are high in immune building flavonoids.

Google explains it well: "Flavonoids are a group of pigments contained in plants and are responsible for the flower and fruit coloration. Flavonoids are present in dietary fruits and vegetables (Macheix et al., 1990). The Citrus peel and seeds are very rich in phenolic compounds, such as phenolic acids and flavonoids. Berries are also very good for your immune system. Choose fresh and always organic.

Tip 3: If you feel fatigued, curl up and rest. The body heals best when resting.

Bonus information: Drink lots of hot liquids, like hot tea and no dairy products except eggs. Gargle with salt water, and for heaven's sake, stop shaking hands with people as this is most likely the way you actually got it in the first place.

Top 14 Natural Anti-Viral Agents:
- Elderberry
- Echinacea
- Garlic
- Green Tea
- Oreganol oil*
- Pau d' arco
- Calendula
- Astragalus Root
- Cat's Claw
- Ginger
- Liquorice Root
- Peppermint
- Zinc inhibits some viruses
- Colloidal Silver has been utilized as a medicine since ancient times to treat scores of ailments, including the bubonic plague.

Remember, Vitamin D3 is actually a hormone. I overheard a doctor telling another doctor that he takes 50K IU's a week and if he feels he is coming down with something he takes 50K a day for 3 days. I am passing this tip on to you.

Please do your own research on these herbs before using.

How to Prevent or Care For a Headache

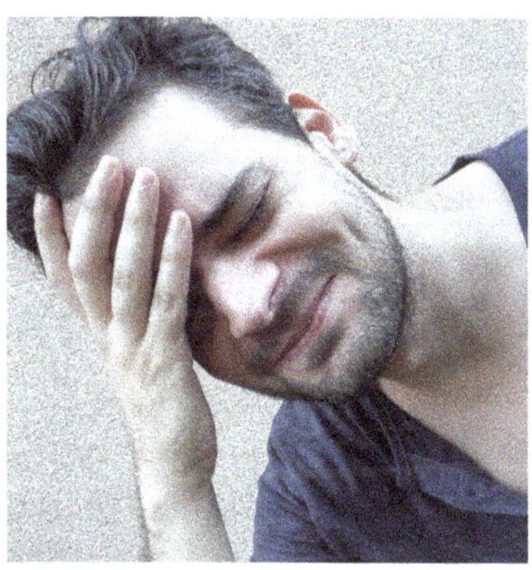

The very first thing to know is that many headaches are caused by mild dehydration. And, if you feel thirsty you are already in mild dehydration. Eye strain is another cause, even poor posture can trigger a headache. Hunger is another trigger.

Tip 1: Drink some water. The best way to keep hydrated is to drink about 1 cup of water every hour–even if you do not feel thirsty. It is said that 65% of people with headaches find relief from drinking water.

Tip 2: Try putting a pencil between your teeth (do not bite down) it may relax the muscles in face and neck and allow your pain to just drain away.

Tip 3: Try sleeping on your back, as other positions may cause some muscles to tighten up, especially in your neck.

Tip 4: Wear sunglasses when in bright sunlight. I know most people know this, however we sometimes just forget.

Tip 5: Peppermint tea can help as well. You can even take a bit of the tea and rub your temples with it. Also, if you have some young living peppermint oil, taking a nice deep breath in can assist in clearing your sinuses.

It is important to note that all essential oils are highly concentrated and be very careful not to get them near your eyes or any soft tissue on your body that could possibly be damaged by the strength of your oil. If you are going to use a medicinal oil one drop in a cup or glass of water or tea is usually the right amount.

Some headaches are brought on from hormones or an imbalance of hormones. Get a hormone saliva test and know where your levels are at. What a difference this can make in your overall health! Hormone headaches can be severe and some are even called migraine.

Contact Sheila Z to order a saliva test.

How to Prevent Diabetes:

How to prevent Type2 Diabetes:

This is a big subject. It is great to cut your carbs way back and give up sugar (easier said than done).

- Remember, pasta turns to sugar, bread turns to sugar. Opt for the sprouted grain bread and remember, usually gluten free has higher carbs than regular bread so be sure and read labels.

- Eat carbs and anything sweet in the first part of the day if you must. High quality protein and fresh organic vegetables can go a long way in prevention.

  - Also Chromium with GTF (chromium picolinate, also Chromium Polynicotinate) is great. 200 mg in the morning is good.

  - Don't eat past 6:PM and stay hydrated.

  - 2 spices that are very good and may keep your blood sugar at normal levels are: True Cinnamon or Ceylon Cinnamon.

  - Cumin. Always opt for organic spices for they are a concentrated form of the herb.

Although, research is still ongoing, early studies report that cumin, among a number of other spices, can have a powerful effect in preventing diabetes by reducing the chances of hypoglycemia. The animals that were tested, showed a sharp decline in hypoglycemia when fed cumin seeds in their diet.

I go into more depth in the *Anatomy of Healing and Wellness* book.

If you would like more information please contact me at: info@Truelife-Solutions.com.

You may also contact me about the
"8 Weeks to Wellness" Program
by going to this web address or
clicking the link on the digital PDF:

https://www.truelife-solutions.com/8-weeks-form/

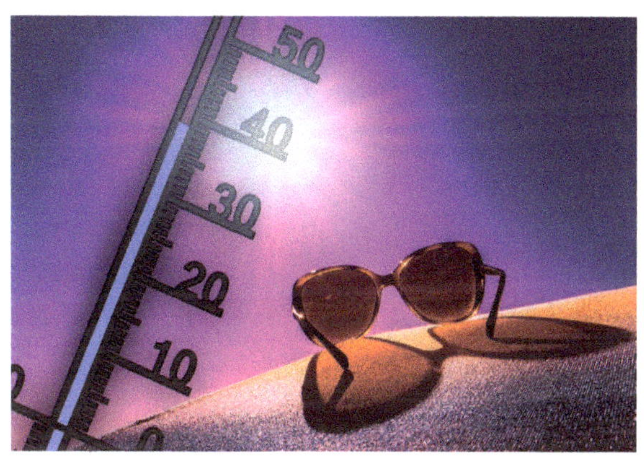

How to Prevent
Over Heating or Heat Stroke:

It is common sense to stay hydrated and when you are in the sun to cover your head. And to be sure you have enough electrolytes.

If you find you are hot and not sweating you are in the beginning stages of a heat stroke.

Tip 1: Put your hands–up to your wrists–in cool or cold water. If you can get your entire body in some cool water this may help.

Tip 2: Eat a pinch of mineral salt.

If you are shivering and hot, nauseous and have mental confusion, you may be a bit late. *Seek medical attention immediately.*

You may be experiencing dehydration even though you have been drinking water. *(Note: real coconut water is a blessing in the heat)* Heat stroke is a serious condition and things can go south quickly, so when we say "seek medical attention immediately,"we mean it! If you have these symptoms get to an emergency room. They will re-hydrate you intravenously. Heat stroke can be life threatening, so please do not take it lightly.

So many times we think, "oh I've just been in the sun too much." This may be true, so always wear a hat when you're in the sun and be sure to take electrolytes with you or coconut water if you're out walking, hiking or sight seeing. If you feel weak DO NOT push yourself to continue. Stop, rest and get to a medical facility.

It takes a few days to recuperate, I can tell you from personal experience. I have had a full blown heat stroke that took weeks to recover from and also more than once had to be re-hydrated in the ER. Take it from me, make it a priority to avoid this.

How to Deal With or Prevent a Yeast Infection

A yeast infection is just that! An overgrowth of yeast caused by Candida, a type of fungus that we all carry in our bodies. This usually shows up in the genital area, however, be aware that if you have fungus on your toes or thrush in your mouth these are all caused by an overgrowth of yeast. You can ask your doctor for an anti-fungal pill and here are some tips you may find interesting.

Tip 1: *Eat lots of True Cinnamon*
Cinnamon has shown an amazing ability to stop medication-resistant yeast infections. This applies to Escherichia coli bacteria and Candida albicans fungus. This study discovered that Cinnamon Oil was one of three leading essential oils effective against Candida. Never, ever get cinnamon near your genitals or face as this oil is strong and will burn.

A second study found that Cinnamon Oil was effective against three strains of Candida, Candida albicans, Candida tropicals, and Candida krusei. Real Ceylon Cinnamon Tea infused with Cinnamon Bark Oil could be an excellent way to fight internal Candida infections and boost your immune system. For topical applications (except genital areas and mucous membranes) 1% Ceylon Cinnamon Leaf Oil mixed with a carrier oil could be an extremely effective treatment option.

Tip 2: Yeast feeds on the sugar in your blood, so a great tip is to really scale down the sugar you are taking in. Yeast does not clear up in a day and can cause all kinds of weird feelings including brain fog and strong cravings.

As the *"8 Weeks to Wellness Program"* has been very successful in dealing with this situation, please feel free to contact me about more in depth information and perhaps the next beginning date for the *"8 Weeks to Wellness Program."*

How to Regain Youthful Skin:

Your skin is the largest organ and many health challenges begin by showing you signs on your skin. This is your body talking to you.

Tip 1: Taking DHEA by mouth seems to increase skin thickness and moisture, and decrease facial "age spots" in elderly men and women.

Tip 2: Your face has many muscles. A few moments every morning of placing your middle finger under the peak of your eyebrows and lightly pushing up while using your muscles to push down. This strengthens your eye brow muscles and may keep your skin from early sagging.

Tip 3: This may sound very weird....but, if you can get your hands on 5PH water this is the best thing for your skin, especially your facial skin. A water store may be able to assist you. I believe the fewer chemicals we put on our faces the better. I don't even use soap of any kind on my face and it seems to have worked out just fine.

Tip 4: Wear a HAT!! Protecting your face from the harsh rays of the sun is one of the best ways to keep that youthful glow even if you are well into your 50's or 60's or beyond.

Sheila Z. Stirling PhD

Using Food as Medicine

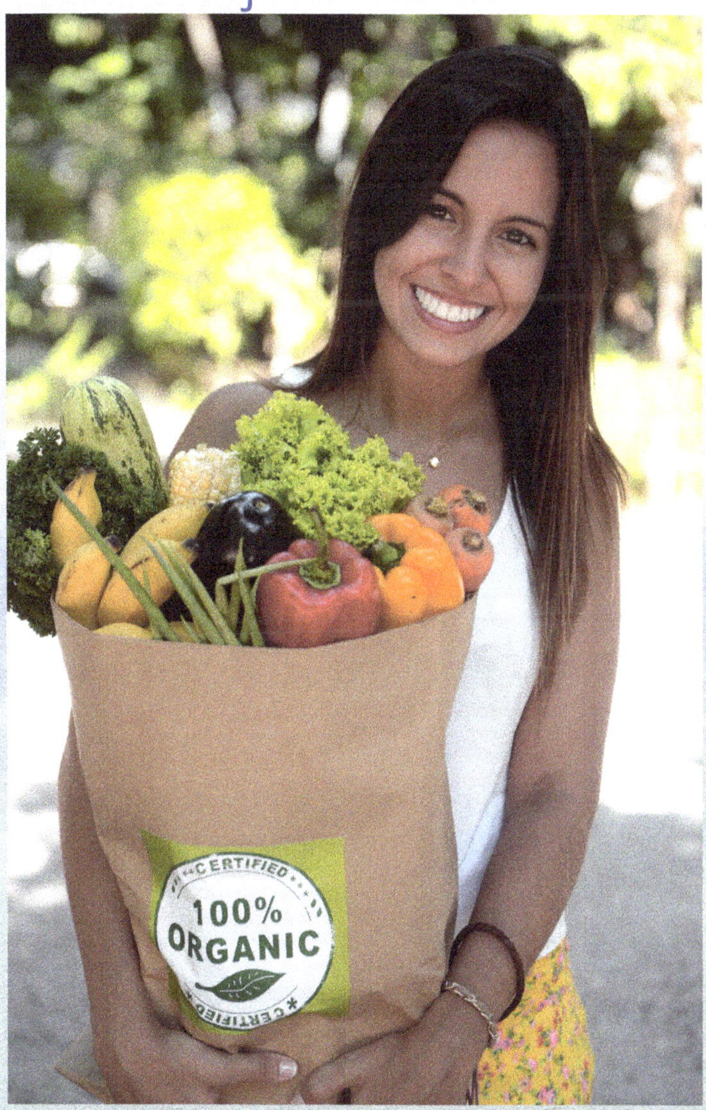

(excerpt from Anatomy of Healing and Wellness)

All through this writing there are hints and tips about food, herbs and supplements being used to help you with your goals for wellness. In this section we will look at specific areas of the body and what foods, herbs and supplements may be your best choice.

Remember, there are other factors when it comes to your vibrant life. Blood type does matter; history and location also play important pieces of the puzzle. Many paths may lead to a given goal. It is becoming very clear that the frequency of the human species is rising, and wonderful paths are opening up everywhere we turn. It is as if the universe has opened up, and sent forth the message that it is time to be well, and understand what unique and beautiful beings we truly are—awakening to the expanded self that awaits within.

That being said, let's dive right in and explore using food as medicine.

Sheila Z. Stirling PhD

Heart Healthy Foods

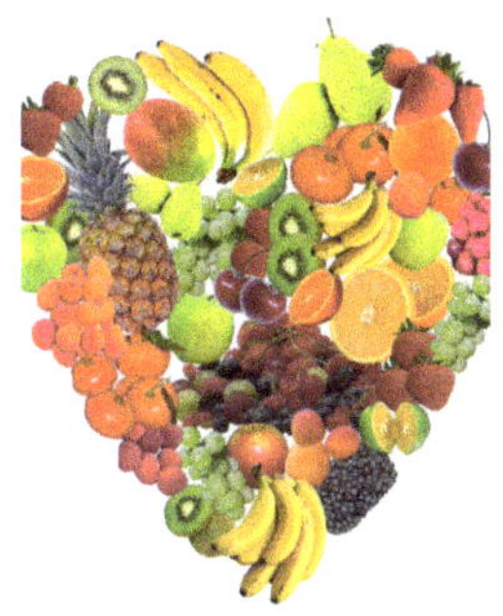

Eating for a healthy heart means filling your plate with fruits and vegetables, paying attention to fiber, eating fish a couple times a week and limiting unhealthy fats like saturated and trans fats, as well as salt. And, although no single food is a cure-all, certain foods have been shown to improve your heart health. Find out how these 12 foods may help lower your risk of heart disease.

Apples

Apples were associated with a lower risk of death from both coronary heart disease and cardiovascular disease, in the Iowa Women's Health Study, which has been tracking 34,000+ women for nearly 20 years.

Finnish researchers studying dietary data collected over 28 years from 9,208 men and women, found that frequent apple eaters had the lowest risk of suffering strokes compared with non-apple eaters. In my programs, we only eat granny smith organic apples as they have a milder effect on blood sugar.

Bananas

One banana has 422 mg—about 12% of your recommended daily dose of potassium. The potassium in bananas helps maintain normal heart function and the balance of sodium and water in the body. Potassium helps the kidneys excrete excess sodium, thereby contributing to healthy blood pressure. This mineral is especially important for people taking diuretics for heart disease, which combat sodium and water retention but, also strip potassium from the body in the process.

Note: Bananas are very high in sugar. If you have, (or your family has) a history of diabetes, please choose other foods to help your heart.

Other good sources of Potassium include:
• Sweet potatoes *(694 mg for one medium),*
• Nonfat yogurt *(579 mg for 1 cup)*
• Spinach *(419 mg for 1/2 cup, cooked)*

Berries

Eating just under a cup of mixed berries daily for eight weeks, was associated with increased levels of *"good"* HDL cholesterol and lowered blood pressure—two positives when it comes to heart health, according to a study of 72 middle-age people published recently in the American Journal of Clinical Nutrition. Included in the mix were strawberries, red raspberries and bilberries (similar to blueberries), as well as other berries more common in Finland *(where the research was conducted).*

The diverse range of polyphenols—a broad class of health-promoting plant compounds that includes anthocyanins and ellagic acid—provided by the mix of berries, is likely responsible for the observed benefits. Polyphenols may increase levels of nitric oxide, a molecule that produces a number of heart-healthy effects.

Green Tea

Some of the strongest evidence of tea's health benefits comes from studies of heart disease. Scientists have found that those who drink 12 ounces (or more) of tea a day, are about half as likely to have a heart attack as non-tea drinkers. Scientists also reported in 2009, that Japanese men who drank a daily cup of green tea significantly lowered their risk of developing gum disease—the more tea, the lower the risk.

The researchers believe that antioxidants called Catechins in green tea are the key. Catechins hamper the body's inflammatory response to the bacteria that cause gum disease. People with gum disease are twice as likely to suffer from heart problems.

Pomegranates

Studies have shown that this fruit may help to reduce the buildup of plaque in arteries and lower blood pressure. Experts believe that the pomegranate's benefits come from its powerful punch of polyphenols—including anthocyanins (found in blue, purple and deep-red foods) and tannins (also found in wine and tea). In a 2008 study, researchers found that; compared with other antioxidant-rich beverages including, blueberry juice, cranberry juice, and red wine; *"pomegranate [juice] naturally has the highest antioxidant capacity," reports David Heber, M.D. PhD., study collaborator and Director of the UCLA Center for Human Nutrition.*

Popcorn

Popcorn delivers polyphenols—antioxidants linked to improving heart health. Gram for gram, popcorn boasts three times more polyphenols than kidney beans (the highest vegetable polyphenol source) and 4 times more than cranberries (the best fruit source), according to recent research out of the University of Scranton. What's more, popcorn is a whole grain—and people who eat plenty of whole grains tend to be leaner and have a lower risk of heart disease than those who don't. *(I found this difficult to believe, but it is true!)*

Pick Fish

Research shows that eating just one or two (4-ounce) servings of fatty fish—salmon, mackerel, rainbow trout or sardines—each week can slash your risk of dying from heart disease by **36%!**

In another study, researchers tracked almost 80,000 women for 14 years and found that those who ate any type of fish, at least twice a week, had a **51%** lower risk of thrombotic stroke (a type caused by clogged arteries) than those who ate fish less than once a month.

A bonus: "The omega 3 fats in fish help reduce inflammation in the arterial walls and keep blood flowing to the brain," *explains Ralph Felder, M.D., PhD., internist and author of The Bonus Years.*

Wine/Alcohol
(It is the picknolgional that is the benefit)
Scientific literature indicates that people who drink moderately are less likely to have heart disease than those who abstain. Drinking in moderation may protect the heart by raising "good" HDL cholesterol, decreasing inflammation and "thinning the blood" (preventing clots that can cause heart attack and stroke).

Moderate drinking also increases estrogen, which protects the heart—a benefit particularly helpful to post-menopausal women whose reduced estrogen levels increase their risk of heart disease.

Remember, 1 drink equals 12 oz of beer, 5 oz of wine or 1.5 oz of liquor.

Grapes (red and purple grapes)
Grapes are rich in health-protecting antioxidants, including resveratrol and flavonoids. So, if you choose not to have alcohol you may still have the benefits by eating grapes. The rich red color of some grapes lets you know this grape is good for your blood and circulation.

Foods Good for the Brain

"The heart and brain are linked by arteries that supply blood, oxygen and nutrients,"says Philip B. Gorelick, M.D., M.P.H., Director of the Center for Stroke Research at the University of Illinois College of Medicine. When plaque builds up and arteries harden, they deprive the heart and brain of blood— and that can lead to a heart attack or stroke. *The good news: A few simple and tasty choices can help protect both your heart and your cranium:*

Foods to Help Avoid Heart Disease, Stroke & Improve Brain Function

For years experts have said, "What's good for the heart, is good for the head." Now, a new statement from the American Heart Association and American Stroke Association underlines the findings that the same plaque buildup in the arteries that causes heart disease can also impact the brain.

Web M.D. had this to say about foods that are good for the brain: "Add these 'superfoods' to your daily diet, and you will increase your odds of maintaining a healthy brain for the rest of your life."

Blueberries

"Brainberries" is what Steven Pratt, MD, (author of *Superfoods Rx: Fourteen Foods Proven to Change*

Your Life) calls these tasty fruits. Pratt, who is also on staff at Scripps Memorial Hospital in La Jolla, Calif., says that, "In animal studies, researchers have found that *blueberries help protect the brain from oxidative stress and may reduce the effects of age-related conditions such as Alzheimer's disease or dementia.*"

Wild Salmon

Deep-water fish, such as salmon, are rich in omega 3 essential fatty acids, which are essential for brain function.

Nuts and Seeds

"Nuts and seeds are good sources of Vitamin E," says Pratt, explaining that higher levels of Vitamin E correspond with less cognitive decline as you get older. *Add an ounce a day of walnuts, hazelnuts, Brazil nuts, filberts, almonds, cashews, peanuts, sunflower seeds, sesame seeds, flax seed, and un-hydrogenated nut butters such as peanut butter, almond butter, and tahini. Raw or roasted doesn't matter. (Please note that cashews are actually a bean and so not permitted on my programs).*

Avocados

Avocados are almost as good as blueberries in promoting brain health. "I don't think the avocado gets its due. True, the avocado is a fatty fruit, but, it's a mono-unsaturated fat, which contributes to healthy blood flow; and healthy blood flow means a healthy brain," says Dr. Kulze. An avocado a day will also keep the doctor away, just like a green apple.

Whole Grains

Whole grains such as oatmeal, whole-grain breads, and brown rice can reduce the risk for heart disease. Every organ in the body is dependent on blood flow. If you promote cardiovascular health, you're promoting good flow to the organ system, which includes the brain. While wheat germ is not technically a whole grain, it also goes on Dr. Kulze's "superfoods" list because in addition to fiber, it has Vitamin E and some Omega 3's.

Kulze suggests: ½ cup of whole-grain cereal, 1 slice of bread two-three times day, or 2 tablespoons of wheat germ a day.

(If you are on the 8 Weeks to Wellness Program or other targeted eating regiment you may be asked to cut the amount of whole grains suggested in this statement)

Older Adults:

Eat Your Antioxidants!

People who eat more brightly colored fruits and leafy vegetables have less cognitive decline than those who don't; antioxidants in produce may mop up free radicals and protect neurons from damage.

Food solutions:

- Berries and other fruits, greens and turmeric (which contains curcumin).

- Pour a Glass of red wine
  Red wine contains compounds called polyphenols

that help lower cholesterol and blood pressure and prevent blood clots.

Research suggests one polyphenol; Resveratrol, may also improve blood flow to the brain and reduce stroke risk. "Resveratrol makes the blood cells less sticky and thus thins out the blood, which prevents dangerous blood clots." Despite the health boons, if you don't drink, don't.

Foods that Lower Cholesterol:

Mono-unsaturated & Polyunsaturated Fats:

- Olive Oil
- Peanut Oil
- Peanuts
- Olives
- Avocados

are healthier fats and are the most powerful thing you can consume to achieve a drastic reduction in your LDL cholesterol.

Specifically, a diet high in olive and sunflower oil, that contains 12.9% saturated fat, 15.1% mono-unsaturated fat, and 7.9% polyunsaturated fat can achieve an 18% reduction in LDL cholesterol versus people on a diet higher in saturated fat.

Bran (Oat, Rice)

Bran (particularly oat bran) has been proven effective in lowering LDL cholesterol levels. Add bran to hot cereals and bread. Also, eating whole oatmeal every morning, or switching to whole products like brown rice, can help you get more bran in your diet and lower your cholesterol numbers by 7-14%.

Flax Seeds

Up to 50 grams of flax seed a day has been shown to reduce LDL cholesterol in healthy young adults by up to 8%, and 38 grams of flax seeds per day reduced LDL cholesterol by 14% in people with high cholesterol (hypercholesterolemia).

In both studies the flax seeds were consumed in a muffin, or other bread product. Flax seeds are easily incorporated in baked goods, as well as added to hot cereals like oatmeal. Try some in a vegetable smoothie. It's very tasty. 50 gr = 1.7 oz about and that is about 3 Tbs.

Garlic

Studies have shown that less than half a clove (900mg) of raw garlic a day can lower cholesterol by 9-12%. Raw garlic is best, and can be added to olive oil salad dressings, or as a garnish on soups and sandwiches.

Almonds

Several studies report that eating up to half a cup of almonds can reduce cholesterol levels by up to 10%. In a dose response study it was found that a quarter cup of almonds reduces cholesterol by 5% and half a cup causes the full 10% reduction.

As almonds are a high calorie food, it is not recommended that you eat more than half a cup. Almonds are great as a snack, or as an addition to breakfast cereals like oatmeal. *There is a catch! Please eat blanched almonds as the skin of the almond is a mild toxin.*

Here is one explanation from google:
"Bitter almonds are from a variety of regular, sweet almonds. Bitter almonds contain traces of prussic acid—also known as hydrocyanic acid—in its raw state. Hydrocyanic acid is a solution of hydrogen cyanide and water. The byproduct is an organic version of the well-known poison, cyanide. Bitter almonds may yield 4–9 mg of hydrogen cyanide per almond and contain 42 times higher amounts of cyanide than the trace levels found in sweet almonds.

Lycopene Foods

Lycopene is a carotenoid pigment responsible for giving fruits and vegetables their red color, and is found in tomatoes, watermelon, and various other high lycopene foods.

Studies are conflicting as to whether lycopene reduces LDL cholesterol or not. Some studies report a 10-17% reduction while other studies find no difference. Despite this difference, lycopene is thought to generally promote heart health whether it lowers LDL cholesterol or not.

Please keep in mind; *tomatoes are a night shade and all night shades promote inflammation.* Because, we now know that inflammation may be a root cause of disease, we do NOT eat any tomatoes in the *8 Weeks to Wellness Program.*

So, use your best judgment and just say **NO** to foods that promote inflammation.

Walnuts and Pistachios

Numerous studies report a reduction in cholesterol with consumption of walnuts or pistachios. This is especially true when the fats from the nuts replace consumption of other high cholesterol fats. Consuming around 30 grams of walnuts, or having the nuts be about 20-30% of total caloric intake is necessary to achieve the cholesterol lowering benefits.

A One ounce (30-grams) serving of walnuts is about 14 halves. 9 whole walnuts provides the following nutrients: Calories: 185. Water: 4% Protein: 4.3 grams.

Whole Barley

Like the bran from oats and rice, barley reduces cholesterol 7–10%, particularly when it is used as a substitute for wheat products. Barley can easily substitute wheat in the form of barley noodles, barley flour, or whole pearl barley.

Dark Chocolate and Plant Sterols

The plant sterols and cocoa flavanols in dark (non-milk) chocolate have been shown to reduce cholesterol by 2-5%. Further, plant sterols (phytosterols), found in all plants, and particularly plant oils have been shown to lower LDL cholesterol by up to 16%. However, this reduction is largely due to inhibiting absorption of cholesterol, and would not have a large effect if you consumed little or no cholesterol.

Green Tea

Green Tea has long been a staple in East Asia where it is believed to wash oil (fat) out of the body. Studies suggest that this may be true, *as green tea can lower cholesterol by 2-5%.* Green tea without sugar also has few calories typically.

Side note: Having a cup of warm liquid, like water will also help to wash the fats out of the body. After every meal my mother would have a cup of English black tea. Did it help her to live to 96?… a distinct possibility.

What Lowers Blood Pressure?
Ginger

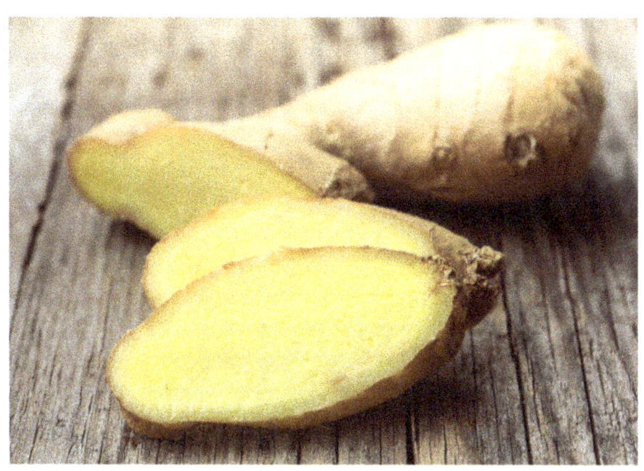

Ginger is one of the ancient, most revered medicines of India and Asia. The list of conditions for which it is used is so long that it might prompt skepticism.

How can one herb affect so many seemingly different diseases?

Here's how this alternative medicine works:
Ginger is not often used by the majority of Americans, even though it commonly appears in the kitchens of countries across the globe. With so many healthy properties to it, it makes sense to start adding this to more of your dishes, or to start brewing a daily glass of ginger tea.

It's easy enough to make ginger tea:
Cut a two-inch cube of ginger (rhizome) into slices and simmer them in one cup of water on low heat for 10 minutes. Cover the pot while cooking to retain as many volatile constituents as possible. Remove the slices, and sip the remaining liquid before a meal. Eat the slices after drinking the tea.

Drink 3 cups of tea per day, one before each meal. Adding lemon is a way to make it taste better and get more benefits from it.

The part of ginger we use is not actually the root, as one might guess from the way it looks. It's actually the rhizome, (or underground stem)—the spicy, aromatic compounds in the rhizome—that impart the medicinal activity to ginger. It is relatively susceptible to heat and oxygen, so tread gingerly when making medicine from this herb. ***Do not refrigerate***, even after it is cut. A dark cool place is best. Use within 2 to 3 weeks for optimal effects.

Prevention & Wonders of Ginger

Fights Cancer:

There are particular cancers that ginger has been shown to help treat, including ovarian cancer. Research has proven that ginger can act to literally obliterate ovarian cancer cells. Even more promising is that the cells actually end up killing and attacking themselves. This is good news for those that already have cancer, and reason enough to start having more ginger show up in your diet if you're currently cancer-free.

Help with Irritable Bowel Syndrome:

Those suffering from IBS will be happy to note that getting more ginger should spell relief from the symptoms of this condition. The interesting thing is, that it doesn't seem to matter how you get the ginger into your system—whether including more ginger root in your cooking, taking ginger supplements, or brewing ginger tea—they all seem to have a calming effect on the bowels and digestive system.

Protections Against Alzheimer's Disease:

If Alzheimer's runs in your family, or you are just worried about coming down with this debilitating disease, you should think about incorporating more ginger into your diet and daily routine. Research has shown that ginger helps to slow down the loss of brain cells that is typically a precursor to Alzheimer's. By protecting and preserving these cells, you are prolonging the amount of good years you have being alert and coherent, and aware of your surroundings.

Maintain Normal Blood Circulation:
Ginger contains chromium, magnesium and zinc which can help to improve blood flow, as well as help prevent chills, fever, and excessive sweat.

Remedies for Motion Sickness:
Ginger is a known effective remedy for the nausea associated with motion sickness. The exact reason is unknown, but in a study of Naval cadets, those given ginger powder suffered less.

Weight Loss & Ginger:
It stimulates the appetite: If you have a sluggish digestive system and find that you need to get your digestive fires going before a meal, ginger can help. It may be the case that you don't produce enough stomach acid, and ginger can act as an appetite stimulant, getting your digestive juices revved up so that you are able to digest your meal better. Improper digestion of foods leaves them fermenting in your digestive tract, and can contribute to weight gain.

Relieves Tired Muscles:
The sort of muscle tiredness you get after strength training, is the type that ginger works best on. This means that your muscles will recover better and allow you to take part in cardio workouts on your off days. It means you'll be more likely to be more active, instead of being out of commission on the days following

your weight lifting workouts. Increased lean muscle mass generally equates to natural weight loss as you burn calories around the clock.

Helps Manage Glucose Levels:
Research out of Australia suggests that ginger can help keep blood glucose levels in check. This is important because these levels have a direct impact on weight loss and weight gain, as well as how energetic or lethargic you feel throughout the day. If you've noticed that you get a midday crash, it's likely due to your blood sugar levels, and adding ginger to your lunch might help you stay focused and on task. This is an *all-natural alternative* to products like "5-Hour Energy."

Helps the Body Absorb Nutrients:
When you're trying to lose weight, getting the right nutrients is essential. But, if your body is overweight and not used to getting the nutrients it needs, it may have become used to not getting the required Vitamins and now it doesn't properly absorb them. More ginger means that you'll be better absorbing the sort of nutrients that will help you in your pursuit and get you better results more quickly with the same amount of effort. Ginger stimulates gastric and pancreatic enzyme secretion, and this is why it helps the body absorb better.

Helps with Morning Sickness:
Pregnant women might want to opt for more ginger intake when they are suffering from bouts of morning sickness. The ginger acts as a calming agent. And, when compared to a placebo, it came

through with shining colors in clinical tests. It's always fun when an all-natural remedy gets backed by scientific research. It's as if science is finally figuring out that natural herbs and foods have great value.

Cold and Flu Prevention:

Ginger has been used for thousands of years as a natural treatment for colds and flu in Asia. The University of Maryland Medical Center states that; "To treat cold and flu symptoms in adults, steep 2 tablespoons of freshly shredded or chopped ginger root in hot water, two to three times a day."

Combats Stomach Discomfort:

Ginger is ideal in assisting digestion, thereby improving food absorption and avoiding possible stomach aches.

Ginger also appears to reduce inflammation in a similar way to aspirin and ibuprofen.

Reduces Arthritic Inflammation:

The anti-inflammatory nature of ginger means that it can help with a host of inflammation-based conditions and diseases. Not least of which is arthritis, which millions of American suffer from, with millions more diagnosed each year as the baby boomer population grows older. There is even a bit of a pain relief characteristic to ginger, which is welcomed news to those that don't want to take a pill every day to relieve pain.

Opens Up Inflamed Airways:

If you have asthma you have likely been scouring the Internet for ways to help open up your airways that don't involve taking steroid-based medications. Ginger has been shown to open up airways by reducing inflammation, and it can also relieve any pain symptoms caused by the problem. This may not solve your asthma condition on its own, but it can be used as part of a comprehensive approach.

Improves Circulation:

Ginger gets the blood in your body flowing, which will give you a feeling of having more energy, and can help you with any feelings of sluggishness or fatigue. It's a great thing to drink if you live in a cold climate, because it will provide the sort of warmth you're really after, the kind that comes from the inside and radiates out. This is because it is opening your pores and getting your overall circulation functioning better.

Precautions:

Ginger is extremely safe. Some people have trouble tolerating its spiciness, but most tend to adapt if they keep taking it. Some concern has been raised because ginger may block platelets from sticking together and cause bleeding, but there have been no cases reported of bleeding in people taking ginger. However, do not take ginger with blood thinners without first consulting your health care professional. Ginger is safe to use for short-term use (a few days).

What Helps to Lower Homocysteine?

What are the symptoms of elevated homocysteine?
There are no symptoms.

What are the causes of elevated homocysteine?

An inadequate intake of B Vitamins, as well as genetic factors that affect the body's absorption and use of folic acid, can lead to elevated homocysteine levels. If this is the case, your intake of folate has to be higher than the RDA of 400 mcg.

Other contributors to elevated homocysteine levels include stress and coffee consumption. The more coffee you drink, the higher your homocysteine levels are likely to be. The stress induced neuro-transmitters, epinephrine and nor-epinephrine are metabolized in the liver via a process that uses methyl groups. This can also increase the need for folic acid. In addition, elevated homocysteine levels may be due to low levels of thyroid hormone, kidney disease, psoriasis and some medications.

What is elevated homocysteine?

Homocysteine is an amino acid and breakdown product of protein metabolism; that when present in high concentrations, has been linked to an increased risk of heart attacks and strokes. *Elevated homocysteine levels are thought to contribute to plaque formation by damaging arterial walls.* High levels may also act on blood platelets and increase the risks of clot formation; however, whether high levels of homocysteine actually cause cardiovascular disease has yet to be agreed upon.

In addition, *some evidence suggests that people with elevated homocysteine levels have twice the normal risk of developing Alzheimer's disease.* Blood levels of homocysteine tend to be highest in people who eat a lot of animal protein and consume few fruits and leafy vegetables, which provide the folic acid and other B Vitamins that help the body rid itself of homocysteine. In addition to the dietary connection, homocysteine is also produced in the body from another amino acid—methionine.

One of methionine's main functions is to provide methyl groups for cellular reactions. A methyl group is a chemical fragment consisting of one carbon and three hydrogen atoms. When methionine donates a methyl group for a cellular reaction, it becomes homocysteine. Typically, homocysteine then receives another methyl group from either folic acid or Vitamin B6 to regenerate methionine. The relationship, if any, between homocysteine levels and heart disease risk remains controversial. [bembu.com/ginger-benefits] howstuffworks.com

Ways to lower homocysteine:
To lower homocysteine levels, Dr. Andrew Weil recommends increasing your intake of B Vitamins, particularly folate, and moderating stress. The richest food sources of folate *(the form of folic acid*

found in food) are green vegetables, orange juice *(real and fresh orange juice)* and beans. Dr. Weil also recommends taking a multivitamin that gives you 400 micro grams of folic acid in addition to what you might get from your diet. *(Some people might absorb this Vitamin better in supplement form, which Dr. Weil considers good insurance.)*
To reduce stress, Dr. Weil advises; practicing breathing exercises, meditation and mind-body exercises such as yoga.

Reducing foods high in animal protein can also help lower homocysteine levels. For optimum health, Dr. Weil recommends an anti-inflammatory diet, which limits total protein intake to between 80 and 120 grams (three to four ounces) daily, and emphasizes protein sources such as fish, beans, whole soy and dairy products.

I agree with this and go a step further. When we limit meat to once a week or less and use other sources of high protein foods we also enhance the over all function of our body.

Foods that Lower Blood Sugar:

Avocados

Don't let the fat content of avocados fool you—they're still good for you! Avocados are full of mono-unsaturated fat, the kind that helps slow the release of sugars into the bloodstream, prompting less insulin release.

Blueberries

A ground-breaking study published in the Journal of Nutrition in 2010 found; a daily dose of the bio-active ingredients from blueberries, increases sensitivities to insulin and may reduce the risk of developing diabetes in at-risk individuals.

Cherries

Cherries contain naturally occurring chemicals called anthocyanins, which could help lower blood sugar levels in people with diabetes. A study published in the Journal of Agricultural and Food Chemistry found; anthocyanins could reduce insulin production by 50%. Anthocyanin-loaded cherries may also protect against heart disease and cancer.

Chia Seeds

This ancient gluten-free grain stabilizes blood sugar, manages the effects of diabetes, improves insulin sensitivities, and aids symptoms related to metabolic syndrome. Adults may take up to two tablespoons (or 15 grams) of Chia seeds per day. Chia seeds also carry about 5 grams of fiber per tablespoon and about 3,000 mg of Omega 3's … a super food for sure!

Cinnamon

A 2003 study in the journal, *Diabetes Care*, showed that cinnamon may cause muscle and liver cells to respond more readily to insulin, thereby improving weight loss. Better response to insulin means better blood sugar balance, and therefore, less insulin released into your body.

Ceylon Cinnamon also seems to reduce several risk factors for cardiovascular disease, including high blood sugar and levels of triglycerides, LDL ("bad") cholesterol, and total cholesterol. *Just ½ teaspoon a day for 20 days is enough to improve your insulin response and lower blood sugar by up to 20%!*

You can get this true cinnamon at the herb store. Remember, quality counts in these matters. I personally have about 6gr. per day—that is about one teaspoon.

Eggs

A study published in 2008 in the *International Journal of Obesity* found overweight and obese people given two eggs a day for breakfast *lost 65% more weight* than those eating a similar breakfast without eggs. The researchers said eating eggs may control hunger by reducing the post-meal insulin response, and control appetite by preventing large fluctuations in both glucose and insulin levels.

Olive oil

Olive oil, rich in the same mono-unsaturated fat found in avocados, prevents not only belly fat accumulation, but also insulin resistance.

Spices

According to a 2005 animal study published in the *Journal of Medicinal Food*; a food-seasoning spice mixture containing various spices improved metabolism of both glucose and cholesterol, reducing blood sugar, and insulin levels.

Fenugreek Seed & Turmeric

Both of these particularly, are anti-diabetic, but in some studies **cumin seed, ginger, mustard, curry leaf, and coriander** also show diabetes-fighting properties.

Vinegar

Vinegar has been found to blunt blood sugar and insulin increases, as well as heighten the sensation of fullness after a higher-carbohydrate meal.

Arizona State University study found; people who started a meal with a vinegar drink enjoyed better blood sugar and insulin profiles following meals.

The blood sugar–balancing effect of vinegar seems to work even better in people with pre-diabetes compared to people with normal insulin sensitivities. Look for white or apple cider vinegar, but, look out for balsamic—it contains more sugar.

Iron

Got iron? 10% of women are anemic, and new studies show that being even mildly iron-deficient affects learning, memory, and attention. Luckily, restoring iron levels to normal also restores cognitive function.

Food solutions for Iron deficiency:
Dark leafy greens, beans, meat or soy. Organic of course.

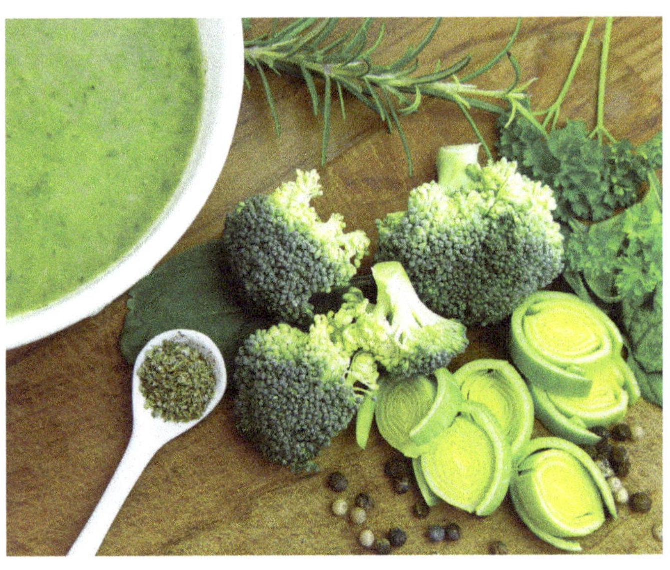

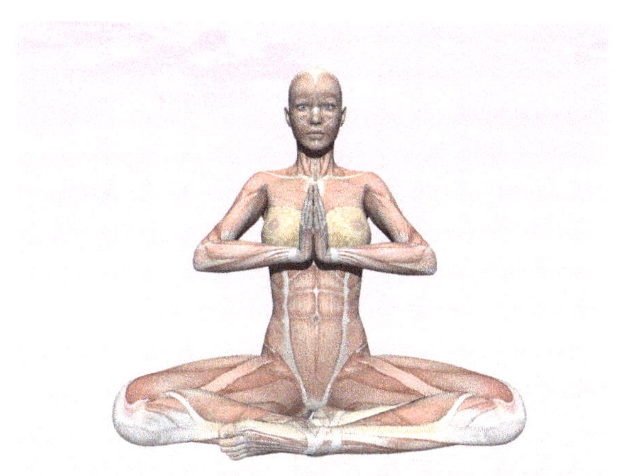

Foods that help Balance Hormones:

Whatever you're eating is either helping hormonal production, or causing unpredictable imbalances. The human body needs a balance of all three macro nutrients: carbohydrates, protein, and especially fat.

Fat is one of the most crucial elements for hormonal balance. For years, we've been told that fat-free is good, while cholesterol and saturated fat are bad. *This is a dangerous lie*. Healthy fat is the raw material that we need to produce and maintain proper hormone function.

Here's why:

Hormones are produced using certain fatty acids and cholesterol. So, if we're missing these nutrients, hormone problems arise simply because the body doesn't have the nutrients it needs to make them.

Our body needs certain fats for rebuilding cells and stabilizing hormones. This is especially important for the female reproductive system.

How to Eat for Hormonal Balance:

Basing your meals off clean protein, hormone balancing healthy fats, antioxidant-rich vegetables, and healing herbs will help your body thrive.

Choose one food from each category
for an easy, hormone balancing,
skin healing meal.

Category 1:
Hormone-balancing Clean protein:
- Soaked or sprouted nuts
- Wild caught fish
- Beans
- Pasture-raised eggs
- Seeds
- Quinoa
- Lentils
- Organic pasture-raised, grass-fed chicken, turkey, beef, bison, elk

Category 2:
Hormone-balancing healthy fats:
- Coconut Oil
- Egg Yolks
- Avocado

- Nuts and seeds
- Raw Butter/Ghee

Why the Above Mentioned Items?

Coconut oil

Coconut oil (and all coconut products for that matter) contains lauric acid, which is incredibly healing to the skin and extremely beneficial for hormonal production. It also kills bad bacteria and viruses in the body, provides a quick source of energy, is easy to digest, and speeds up metabolism.

Avocados

They're rich in healthy fats that help our body absorb and use nutrients. They are also full of fiber, potassium, magnesium Vitamin E, B-Vitamins, Folic acid–all essential for maintaining hormonal balance in the body.

Raw Butter/Ghee

They provide a rich source of fat-soluble Vitamins A, D, E and K2. These nutrients are key building blocks for hormonal production. Butter provides great amounts of short and medium-chain fatty acids, which support immune function, boost metabolism and have anti-microbial properties; meaning, they fight against bad bacteria and viruses in the body.

Egg yolks

They're rich in many vitamins & minerals including:
- A, D, E, B2, B6, B9

- Phosphorous
- Iron
- Potassium
- Calcium
- Choline

These all contribute to a healthy reproductive system, hormonal balance, and healthy skin. The Choline and iodine in egg yolks are also crucial for making healthy thyroid hormones.

Nuts and Seeds

Soaked nuts and seeds, olives and olive oil, fermented cod liver oil, hemp seed oil, flax-seed oil, and raw cultured dairy products.

Antioxidant-Rich Vegetables

Look for anything dark green:

- Asparagus
- Cabbage
- Kale
- Broccoli
- Cucumbers
- Cilantro
- Collard greens
- Spinach

Opt for Brightly Colored Veggies:

- Green red, yellow, and orange
- Bell peppers *(this is a night shade)*
- Tomatoes *(this is a night shade)*
- Red cabbage
- Carrots
- Red/white onions

Don't over look Starchy Vegetables:
* Sweet potatoes
* Artichokes
* Spaghetti squash
* Butternut squash
* Yucca
* Turnips
* Beets

Here a few herbs that are also known for their hormone balancing properties:
* Cinnamon
* Cumin
* Turmeric
* Garlic
* Cayenne
* Ginger

Please see more detail on these herbs in the herb section.

If your body has the nutrients it needs to be in hormonal balance, it will be. You'll experience glowing skin, stable moods, fertility, and consistent energy. Our bodies have an incredible ability to heal and be in balance, when given the nutrients they need to flourish.

Foods Good for the Liver:

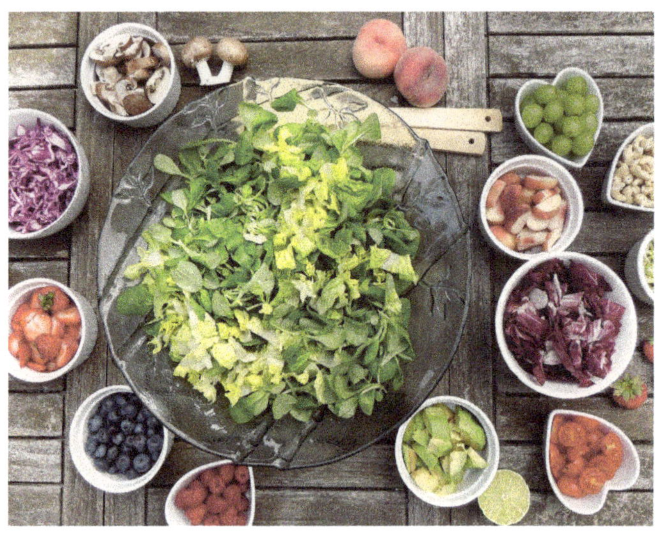

Garlic

Just a small amount of this pungent white bulb has the ability to activate liver enzymes that help your body flush out toxins. Garlic also holds high amounts of allicin and selenium, two natural compounds that aid in liver cleansing.

Grapefruit

High in both Vitamin C and antioxidants, grapefruit increases the natural cleansing processes of the liver. A small glass of freshly-squeezed grapefruit juice will help boost production of the liver detoxification enzymes that help flush out carcinogens and other toxins.

Beets and Carrots

Both are extremely high in plant-flavonoids and beta-carotene; eating beets and carrots can help stimulate and improve overall liver function.

Green Tea

This liver-loving beverage is full of plant antioxidants known as Catechins,a compound known to assist liver function. Green tea is not only delicious, it's also a great way to improve your overall diet.

Leafy Green Vegetables

One of our most powerful allies in cleansing the liver, leafy greens can be eaten raw, cooked, or juiced. Extremely high in plant chlorophyll, greens suck up environmental toxins from the blood stream. With their distinct ability to neutralize heavy metals, chemicals and pesticides, these cleansing foods offer a powerful protective mechanism for the liver.

Incorporate leafy greens into your diet such as:
- Bitter Gourd
- Arugula
- Dandelion Greens
- Spinach
- Mustard Greens
- Chicory

This will help increase the creation and flow of bile, the substance that removes waste from the organs and blood.

Avocados

This nutrient-dense superfood helps the body produce glutathione, a compound that is necessary for the liver to cleanse harmful toxins.

Apples

Apples are high in pectin, and hold the chemical constituents necessary for the body to cleanse and release toxins from the digestive tract. This–in turn–makes it easier for the liver to handle the toxic load during the cleansing process.

Olive Oil

Cold-pressed organic oils such as olive, hemp and flaxseed are great for the liver, when used in moderation. They help the body by providing a lipid base that can suck up harmful toxins in the body. In this way, it takes some of the burden off the liver in terms of the toxic overload many of us suffer from.

Alternative Grains

It's not only that you need alternative grains like Quinoa, millet, and buckwheat in your diet, it's that if you've got wheat, flour, or other whole grains already in your diet...it's time to make changes. Your liver is your body's filter for toxins, and grains that contain gluten are full of them. A study last year found; that persons who experienced gluten sensitivities also had abnormal liver enzyme test results, and that's just one of many.

Cruciferous Vegetables

Eating broccoli and cauliflower will increase the amount of glucosinolate in your system, adding to enzyme production in the liver. These natural enzymes help flush out carcinogens, and other toxins, out of our body which may significantly lower risks associated with cancer.

Lemons & Limes

These citrus fruits contain very high amounts of Vitamin C, which aids the body in synthesizing toxic materials into substances that can be absorbed by water. Drinking freshly-squeezed lemon or lime juice in the morning helps stimulate the liver.

Walnuts

Holding high amounts of the amino acid arginine, walnuts aid the liver in detoxifying ammonia. Walnuts are also high in glutathione and omega 3 fatty acids, which support normal liver cleansing actions. Make sure you chew the nuts well (until they are liquified) before swallowing.

Cabbage

Much like broccoli and cauliflower, eating cabbage helps stimulate the activation of two crucial liver detoxifying enzymes that help flush out toxins. Try eating more kimchi, coleslaw, cabbage soup and sauerkraut.

Turmeric

The liver's favorite spice! Try adding some of this detoxifying goodness into your next lentil stew or veggie dish for an instant liver pick-me-up. Turmeric helps boost liver detox, by assisting enzymes that actively flush out dietary carcinogens.

Other foods that assist the liver include:
• Artichoke
• Kale
• Asparagus
• Brussel sprouts
Always cook or steam asparagus.

"Eating the foods listed above is a great way to help keep your liver functioning properly"
Dr. Edward F. Group III, DC, ND, DACBN, DCBCN, DABFM

Foods that are good for the Pancreas:

When you want a healthy, happy pancreas, you've got plenty of foods to choose from.

Try these, for instance:
• Fish, eggs, and poultry
• D-fortified cereals and dairy

• *Onion and Arugula*
They're tasty on sandwiches and pack special cancer-clubbing flavonols. Seems these two veggies not only add tasty, gourmet-style crunch food, but also fill you up with potent nutrients thought to help thwart pancreatic cancer.

In an 8-year study, people who consumed the highest levels of 3 powerful flavonols— *Kaempferol, Quercetin and Myricetin— reduced their risk of pancreatic cancer by 23%*—no doubt due to the fact that this super trio of flavonols helps quell oxidative stress, a cell-damaging process that, left unchecked, may pave the way for cancer and other bad health news. Onions and certain leafy greens like Arugula are one way to get these particular flavonols.

- *Kaempferol:*
    - Kale
    - Swiss chard
    - Endive
    - Raw Spinach
    - White Beans
- *Quercetin:*
    - Asparagus
    - Green Apples
    - Buckwheat
    - Tea

- *Myricetin:*
    - Fennel
    - Blueberries
    - Cranberries
    - Carob Flour

Health Benefits of Sauerkraut:

Sauerkraut delivers some solid health benefits, including providing fiber and a significant amount of Vitamins C and K. It also boosts your energy and immune system with iron. In spite of the positives, you should limit the amount you eat. Since it's fermented with salt, sauerkraut is high in sodium. One cup contains 39% of your recommended daily intake.

Potential Probiotic Benefits:
As cabbage ferments to produce sauerkraut, it produces a diverse population of live bacteria. These probiotics replenish the good bacteria in your gut and help inhibit the growth of bad bacteria. They may also boost your immune system, synthesize B Vitamins and relieve diarrhea caused by taking antibiotics. However, heat kills live bacteria.
If you cook it, or buy pasteurized sauerkraut, you won't benefit from the probiotics. Look for fresh sauerkraut, or brands that add live bacteria back into the product after pasteurization. If you have had gall stones, it is said by drinking one cup of sauerkraut juice once, or twice a week, you can ward off future stones.

The health benefits derived from pickling vegetables were already well-known to early civilizations. Historical evidence suggests laborers on the Great Wall of China consumed a version of the pickled cabbage dish 2,000 years ago.

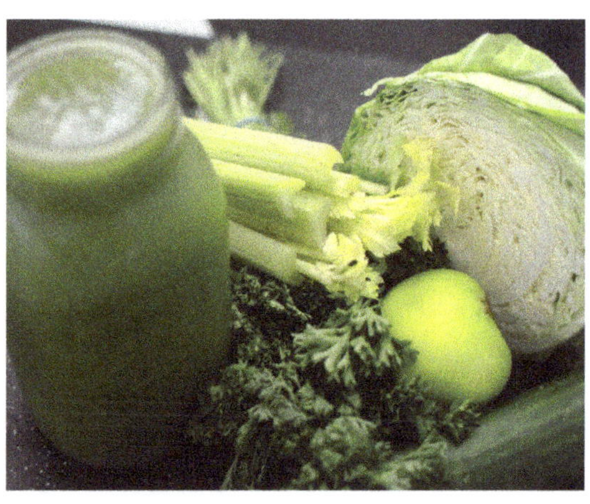

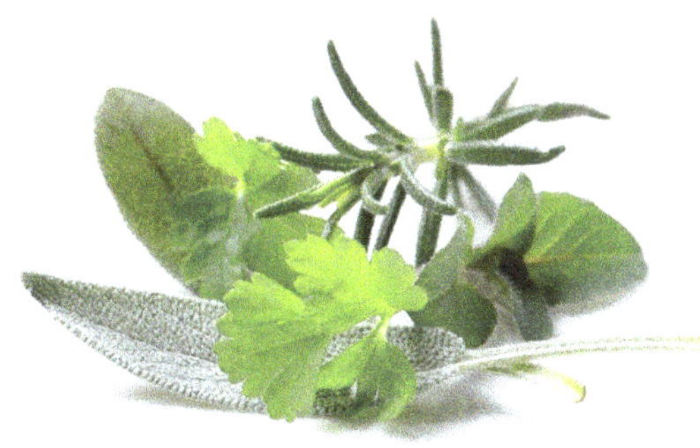

Lets Talk Herbs:

Most herbs you buy in a grocery store have been through a process they call irradiated. This means the herb has been subjected to high temperatures in order to kill any unknown substance. Unfortunately, this also kills most, if not all, medicinal benefits of the herb or spice. Please venture to a herbal store to purchase high quality herbs and spices. Remember, quality does matter.

Medicinal herbs have been used successfully for thousands of years in most countries worldwide. Here are 10 main herbs I always keep on hand. Please be reminded; if you are using herbs or spices, always consider the quality. Not all spices are equal. Cinnamon is a perfect example of that. Buy organic true Cinnamon. Seek out an herb shop in your area. Buy non-irradiated spices and herbs.

There are so many more herbs to consider. Please email me with questions on a specific herb.

The Health Benefits of:
Andrographis

Andrographis Paniculata is a bitter tasting annual plant, referred to as the "King of Bitters." It has white-purple flowers, and it is native to Asia and India, where it has been valued for centuries for its numerous medicinal benefits. Over the past decade, Andrographis has become popular in America, where it is often used (alone and in combination) with other herbs, for a variety of health purposes.

Mechanism of Action:
According to *Memorial Sloan-Kettering Cancer Center,* the active ingredient in Andrographis is andrographolides. Due to the andrographolides, Andrographis has potent anti-inflammatory and antimalarial properties. It also has antimicrobial properties, meaning it can help to fight off, and prevent infections from harmful micro-organisms such as; viruses, bacteria, and fungi. In addition, Andrographis is a powerful antioxidant, and it can help to prevent free radical-induced damage to your cells and DNA.

Cold and Flu
Scientists have discovered that Andrographis helps to boost the immune system by stimulating the body's production of antibodies and macrophages,

which are large white blood cells that scavenge harmful microorganisms. It is taken for both the prevention and treatment of the common cold, and it is often referred to as Indian Echinacea. It might help lessen the severity of cold symptoms such as sleeplessness, fever, nasal drainage and sore throat.

How to use: From 5 to 6 grams daily of dried powered herb can be placed in a gelatin capsule and taken with a glass of water. 4.5 gr=1 tsp.

Or, place 1 teaspoon of the dried leaf tea in a teapot (or tea infuser) and pour over 1 cup of boiling water. Allow to steep 5-10 minutes; sip before meals. (I put just a bit; ¼ tsp. into warm water and sip before a meal.) It's very bitter!!

Ashwagandha

Ashwagandha, one of the most vital herbs in Ayurvedic healing, has been used since ancient times for a wide variety of conditions, but is most well known for its restorative benefits.

In Sanskrit Ashwagandha means "the smell of a horse," indicating that the herb imparts the vigor and strength of a stallion, and it has traditionally been prescribed to help people strengthen their immune system after an illness.

In fact, it's frequently referred to as "Indian ginseng" because of its rejuvenating properties *(although botanically, ginseng and ashwagandha are unrelated)*. In addition, Ashwagandha is also used to enhance sexual potency for both men and women.

Belonging to the same family as the tomato; Ashwagandha (or Withania somnifera in Latin) is a plump shrub with oval leaves and yellow flowers. It bears red fruit about the size of a raisin. The herb is native to the dry regions of India, northern Africa, and the Middle East, but today is also grown in more mild climates, including in the United States.

How much should I take?
The usual recommended dose is 600 to 1000 mg, twice daily (1 teaspoon). For people who suffer from insomnia and anxiety, having a cup of warm almond milk that contains a teaspoon of powdered Ashwagandha before bedtime is beneficial.

Also called the winter cherry, research shows Ashwagandha may be a promising alternative for cancer treatment and prevention. Ashwagandha seems to show positive effects on the endocrine, cardio, and central nervous systems. It is one herb that could help your body produce its own thyroid hormones.

Ashwagandha also improves the body's ability to fight against disease and is a potent antioxidant. It has also shown to be good for the brain in reducing inflammation. Please consult with your health care professional if you are on medications, always check before you take any supplement or herbs.

Boswellia

Traditional use of the herb Boswellia has been celebrated for thousands of years. Also known as frankincense, Boswellia was considered so valuable in ancient times that it was one of the choice gifts brought by the Wise Men to Baby Jesus. Boswellia has not been a part of conventional medicine, nor is it one of the most popular herbs in the lay press, but it does have some properties that could provide substantial benefit for many of today's chronic illnesses.

Boswellia has become a popular herb recently for its benefits in fighting inflammation, which involves many processes that the body uses to help heal itself. It is most evident when we sprain an ankle and develop swelling and tenderness. However, inflammation that goes on day after day can lead to chronic problems such as arthritis or cancer. Boswellia appears to have the ability to counteract inflammation.

This anti-inflammatory effect could correlate to benefit many chronic illnesses like arthritis, asthma and inflammatory bowel disease. Boswellia faces the same challenge that many herbs with a history of use face; it is fairly new to the research field.

That being said, there is incoming data that supports Boswellia's role in chronic illness. It has a long history of use in India for arthritis, and research shows that Boswellia in combination with curcumin is helpful for arthritis pain. Asthma is another chronic illness affected by inflammation. Asthma sufferers noted less attacks and better measurable air movement through the lungs when treating with Boswellia.

Ulcerative colitis represents another disease in which the bowels are plagued with chronic inflammation. It too, has had benefit through Boswellia. There is data to suggest that Boswellia can even modify inflammation seen with swelling from cancer of the brain, perhaps with swelling that comes with cancer treatment.34 In fact, Boswellia might have the ability to fight several different types of cancer cells, including brain cancer cells.

While asthma and inflammatory bowel disease could be areas that can benefit from Boswellia treatment, one of the biggest areas of use for Boswellia is arthritis. Dosage tends to be 300-400 mg, three times a day.

For those looking for arthritis treatments, Boswellia is best if used in combination with turmeric, another anti-inflammatory herb and joint tissue supplement like MSM or glucosamine. Boswellia and its early success is quite exciting. It does not quite have the body of literature that turmeric, essential fatty acids, CoQ10 and Vitamin D have, but it could still be useful for many chronic diseases.

It is hard to know exactly why the Wise Men of ancient times valued Boswellia so highly, but it is becoming clear that it does have the ability to help the body in many ways. Inflammation is becoming more recognized as the plague of developed nations everywhere. Diet, exercise and anti-inflammatory supplements like Boswellia might be the best line of defense. Boswellia also known as Indian Frankincense.

Burdock

Have you ever returned from a romp with your dog and found burrs on your clothing and in your pup's fur? Then you've literally come in contact with burdock. Arctium bears its seeds in the form of small spherical burrs, hence the name burdock. Close examination of a burdock burr reveals a small hook on the end of its tiny spikes. These hooks catch on the fur of passing animals or on the clothes of passing people, thus dispersing the plant's seeds. Burdock was the inspiration for Velcro fasteners! But, Burdock is more than just a sticky substance. By using the roots—or in some cases, its leaves and seeds—burdock can be utilized in a number of herbal remedies to aid in digestion and more.

Uses of Burdock

Burdock is a perennial whose roots, leaves, and sometimes its seeds, are used widely in herbal medicine to support liver function and as a cleansing botanical. Like dandelion and yellow dock, burdock roots are bitter, and thus capable of stimulating digestive secretions and aiding digestion. These roots are referred to as "alternative" agents—capable of enhancing digestion and the absorption of nutrients and supporting the elimination of wastes. Any botanical capable of these important actions can attain far-reaching improvements in a variety of complaints.

Burdock seeds and roots may be useful in treating a variety of skin conditions, including acne and dryness, especially when these complaints are due to poor diet, constipation, or liver burden. The liver plays an important role in removing impurities from the blood, producing bile to digest fats, metabolizing hormones, and storing excess carbohydrates, in addition to its other functions. Everything absorbed from the digestive tract goes directly to the liver to be filtered, so, when you eat foods that contain pesticides, preservatives, artificial coloring and the like, you give your liver extra work to do. A high-fat diet also forces your liver to work harder because it must break down the fat with the bile it produces.
Add to this all of the potential toxins to which we are exposed in daily life that the liver must remove from the bloodstream (car exhaust, nicotine, prescription drugs, alcohol, cleaning products, industrial toxins, etc.), and you can see how the liver can become overworked or burdened.

In folk medicine, the seeds of the burdock were compressed to make a mixture that provided relief for measles, arthritis, tonsillitis, throat pain, and viruses like the common cold. Burdock root can also be used to treat gout, rheumatism, ulcers, acne, eczema, and psoriasis. Folk herbalists use it to treat snake bites and those that are afflicted with rabies. They also used dried burdock as a diuretic, diaphoretic, and a blood purifying agent. It purifies the blood by getting rid of dangerous toxins.

Chaga

It is the most powerful sought after mushroom on earth. It's one of the highest—if not the highest—antioxidants in the world and it's documented extensively for having numerous health benefits, but it's publicized mostly as an anti-cancer.

It is also known for de-calcifying the pineal gland. Chaga has demonstrated anti-HIV, antibacterial, anti-malarial, anti-inflammatory and is also antiviral, anti-fungal, antimicrobial. Chaga is an immune system modulator as well as an adaptogen and has the highest level of super-oxide dismutase or (SOD) detected in any food or herb in the world and what that means for you is that it will super charge your immune system, assist in stabilizing free radicals. Free radical damage can lead to cancer.

Chaga is also rich in Vitamin B1 (Thiamine), Vitamin B2 (Riboflavin), Vitamin B3 (Niacin), Vitamin D2 (Ergosterol), Vitamin K and Zinc.37.

The most common use is to make Chaga tea.

Chaga tea can be made from:
1 to 2 teaspoons of Chaga powder in water warmed to 125 degrees.
Let it steep for about 10 min.

People who drink this tea have reported stronger immune systems, lower cholesterol, better mental clarity and even smoother skin. This is one powerful mushroom! (There is about 3 entire pages dedicated to this amazing mushroom in my *Anatomy of Healing and Wellness* book.

Anti-Candida: Chaga promotes and protects the functions of the liver which busily processes Candida toxins. Chaga has properties that help to lower cholesterol, inflammation and blood pressure levels through sterols and triterpenes. Chaga contains B and D Vitamins and lots of protein which promote relief from stress, depression and fatigue which Candida sufferers deal with.

Chlorella

Has been shown to increase the good bacteria in the gastrointestinal (GI) tract, which helps to treat **ulcers, colitis, diverticulosis and Crohn's disease.** It is also used to treat **constipation, Fibromyalgia, high blood pressure and high cholesterol.**

Chlorella has been used to treat cancer and also help protect the body from the effects of cancer radiation treatment. The algae, which is a popular food supplement in Asia, and has been used as energy- producing food for centuries, is often used to prevent, or curb the spread of cancer, enhance immunity, promote a good balance of bacteria in the gut, and lower blood cholesterol.

In Japan, it is traditionally used as a treatment for **duodenal ulcers, gastritis, hypertension, diabetes, hypoglycemia, asthma, and constipation.** More recently, it has been touted as an effective therapy for elevated cholesterol levels, a prophylactic to ward off infections and adjunct treatment for cancer. Chlorella is now used as an adjunct supplement during radiation treatment for cancer. Its abundance of chlorophyll is known to protect the body against ultraviolet radiation. It is a nutrient-dense superfood that contains 60% protein, 18 amino acids (including all the essential amino acids), and various Vitamins and minerals. One of its unique properties is a phytonutrient called CGF.

Chlorella provides all of the dietary essential amino acids in excellent ratios. It is also a reliable source of essential fatty acids that are required for many important biochemical functions, including hormone balance. Chlorella also contains high levels of chlorophyll, beta-carotene and RNA/DNA.

Chlorella is a fresh water, single-celled algae that grows in fresh water. Chlorella emerged over 2 billion years ago, and was the first form of a plant with a well-defined nucleus. Because Chlorella is a microscopic organism, it was not discovered until the late 19th century, deriving its name from the Greek, "chloros" meaning green and "ella" meaning small. In fact, Chlorella contains the highest amount of chlorophyll of any known plant. It is thought to boost the immune system and help fight infection.

More than 20 Vitamins and minerals are found in Chlorella, including iron, calcium, potassium, magnesium, phosphorous, pro-Vitamin A, Vitamins C, B1, B2, B2, B5, B6, B12, E and K, biotin, inositol, folic acid, plus Vitamins C, E and K.

Although the algae grows naturally in fresh water, Chlorella destined for human consumption is generally cultivated outdoors in mineral-rich freshwater ponds under direct sunlight. The entire process from strain maintenance in the laboratory, to harvesting of the final product, is monitored by microbiologists to ensure optimal nutrient value and product purity. It is often combined with other natural green foods such as spirulina, wheat grass, barley greens, and sometimes seaweed.

Chlorella has been the focus of many medical and scientific research projects. Based on very early research, it appears that Chlorella may play a role in **Fibromyalgia, hypertension, or ulcerative colitis and has an effect on the immune system.** More studies are needed to confirm initial findings.

Research conducted in Japan suggests that Chlorella may have anti-tumor activities against **breast cancer.** However, its main use in cancer therapy is to help remove radioactive particles from the body after radiation treatment.

So far, the bulk of evidence for Chlorella's long list of medicinal powers comes from animal studies. Studies in mice have shown that Chlorella vulgaris can protect against the development and spread of cancer, and other rodent studies have shown that it lowers cholesterol and helps organisms get rid of toxic chemicals,such as dioxins.

Cinnamon
(True Cinnamon)

Stomach Bug/Flu:
By far, the best remedy for a horrible stomach bug is Cinnamon. It makes sense because, cinnamon is a powerful anti-bacterial.

Research has shown that Cinnamon is one of the most effective substances against Escherichia coli, Salmonella, and Campylobacter. Another study found Cinnamaldehyde, from Cinnamon Bark Oil in its various forms, is effective against adenovirus. Another reason to have Cinnamon tea infused with Cinnamon Bark Oil that has high levels of Cinnamaldehyde (between 40-50%).

Irritable Bowel Syndrome (IBS):
As a digestive, cinnamon dramatically reduces the uncomfortable feelings associated with IBS—especially the bloating. It does this by killing bacteria and healing infections in the GI tract and enabling

the gastric juices to work normally. A Japanese study apparently showed it to cure ulcers, but this cannot be verified. But, if you do have stomach cramps or upsets, a cup of Cinnamon tea 2-3 times per day will dramatically reduce the pain.

Dandelion Root

The Dandelion root is a very economical herb considering that it is a weed that most of us dig and get rid of! I have been eating it for years.

Dandelion is a great spring tonic for our bodies; it helps the transition from winter to the warmer season, by nourishing and balancing the blood so it will flow better and keep us cooler in the summer season.

Health Benefits of Dandelion Root:

- Widely recognized as a liver tonic, as it nourishes the liver.

- Because of its high iron and zinc content, dandelion root is often used as a treatment for anemia.

- Has mild laxative properties and is often used to help maintain regularity.

- Recognized as a great blood builder and for the liver.

- Aids skin problems as well as detoxifies poisons and toxic waste in the body.

- It is also a mild appetite stimulant; tea made from root and leaves can help relieve digestive problems.

- Dandelion root functions as a mild diuretic. Because potassium is often lost when using a diuretic, dandelion root is often a better choice for a diuretic than synthetic formulas.

- Lowers cholesterol according to some studies. Early results of at least one study show that dandelion root supplements may affect the cholesterol profile in diabetic mice positively, by lowering LDL and triglycerides while increasing HDL.

- Its positive effects on the liver and digestion may help the effectiveness of other Vitamins, minerals and nutrients.

- Dandelion acts as a tonic to the system. It destroys acid in the blood. As it contains organic sodium, it is very good for the deficiency of nutritive salts, and is recognized as a great blood builder and purifier.

Dandelion Root Nutrition:
- Filled with Vitamins A, C, D and B complex.
- Minerals such as zinc, iron and potassium.
- High in calcium and other nutrients.

Milk Thistle

Milk Thistle Benefits:
Milk Thistle is unique in its ability to protect the liver and has no equivalent in the pharmaceutical drug world. In fact, in cases of poisoning with Amanita mushrooms—which destroy the liver—Milk Thistle is the only treatment option. It has been so dramatically effective that the treatment has never been disputed, even by the traditional medical community. Milk Thistle acts in a similar fashion to detoxify other synthetic chemicals that find their way into our bodies, from acetaminophen and alcohol to heavy metals and radiation.

Milk thistle was approved in 1986 as a treatment for **liver disease** and it is widely used to treat **alcoholic hepatitis, alcoholic fatty liver, cirrhosis, liver poisoning and viral hepatitis.** It has also been shown to protect the liver against medications such as acetaminophen, a non-aspirin pain reliever.
The active ingredient, or liver-protecting compound in Milk Thistle is known as silymarin. This substance, which actually consists of a group of compounds called flavonolignands, helps repair liver cells damaged by alcohol and other toxic substances by stimulating protein synthesis. By changing the outside layer of liver cells, it also prevents certain toxins from getting inside. Silymarin also seems to encourage liver cell growth.

It can reduce inflammation (important for people with liver inflammation or hepatitis), and has potent antioxidant effects. Antioxidants are thought to protect body cells from damage caused by a chemical process called oxidation. Milk Thistle is not standardized to an exact amount (as it is made from pure dried natural herbs. Milk Thistle naturally contains about 70 - 80% Silymarin (and many other constituents thought to work in harmony).

This herb benefits adrenal disorders and IBS (Inflammatory Bowel Syndrome), and is used to treat psoriasis (increases bile flow).

Milk thistle has some estrogen-like effects that may stimulate the flow of breast milk in women who are breast-feeding infants. It may also be used to start late menstrual periods. Milk thistle's estrogen-like effect may also have some usefulness for men with prostate cancer.

In animal studies and one small study in humans, Milk Thistle produced modest reductions in total cholesterol. However, these results have not been demonstrated in larger human studies. This herb is a must for cleansing and for anyone with any sort of liver dysfunction or exposure to toxins.

Liver disease from alcohol:

A comprehensive review by the U.S. Agency for Healthcare Research and Quality (AHRQ) recently identified 16 scientific studies on the use of Milk Thistle for the treatment of various forms of liver disease. A European standardized extract of Milk Thistle was used in most of the trials. Problems in study design (such as small numbers of participants, variations in the causes of liver disease, and differences in dosing and duration of Milk Thistle therapy) made it difficult to draw any definitive conclusions.

However, five of seven studies evaluating Milk Thistle for alcoholic liver disease found significant improvements in liver function. Those with the mildest form of the disease appeared to improve the most. Milk Thistle was less effective for those with severe liver disease such as cirrhosis. Cirrhosis is characterized by scarring and permanent, non-reversible damage to the liver. It is often referred to as end-stage liver disease.

Viral hepatitis:

Despite the fact that Milk Thistle is widely used in the treatment of hepatitis (particularly hepatitis C), results from four viral hepatitis studies were contradictory. Some found improvements in liver enzyme activities while others failed to detect these benefits. None of the studies compared Milk Thistle with interferon or other medications for viral hepatitis.

Cancer:

Preliminary laboratory studies also suggest that active substances in Milk Thistle may have anti-cancer effects. One active substance known as silymarin has strong antioxidant properties and has been shown to inhibit the growth of human prostate, breast, and cervical cancer cells in test tubes. Further studies are needed to determine whether Milk Thistle is safe or effective for people with these forms of cancer.

High cholesterol:

One animal study found that silymarin (an active compound in Milk Thistle) worked as effectively as the cholesterol-lowering drug probucol, with the additional benefit of substantially increasing HDL ("good") cholesterol. Further studies in people are needed.

Nettle

Nettle Benefits:

Nettle has been used for centuries to treat allergy symptoms, particularly hay fever which is the most common allergy problem. It contains biologically active compounds that reduce inflammation. Dr. Andrew Weil M.D., author of Natural Health/Natural Medicine says, he knows of nothing more effective than Nettle for allergy relief, and his statement is backed up by studies at the National College of Naturopathic Medicine in Portland, Oregon.

Decongestants, antihistamines, allergy shots and even prescription medications such as Allegra and Claritin treat only the symptoms of allergies and tend to lose effectiveness over a period of time. They can also cause drowsiness, dry sinuses, insomnia and high blood pressure. Nettle has none of these side effects. It can be used on a regular basis and has an impressive number of other benefits most notably as a treatment for prostate enlargement.

Nettle has been studied extensively and has shown promise in treating:

- Alzheimer's disease
- Arthritis
- Asthma
- Bladder infections
- Bronchitis
- Bursitis
- Gingivitis
- Gout
- Hives
- Kidney stones
- Laryngitis
- Multiple Sclerosis
- PMS
- Prostate Enlargement
- Sciatica
- Tendinitis!

Externally it has been used to improve the appearance of the hair, and is said to be a remedy against oily hair and dandruff. In Germany today, Stinging Nettle is sold as an herbal drug for prostate diseases and as a diuretic. It is a common ingredient in other herbal drugs produced in Germany for rheumatic complaints and inflammatory conditions (especially for the lower urinary tract and prostate).

In the United States many remarkable healing properties are attributed to Nettle and the leaf is utilized for different problems than the root.

The leaf is used here **as a diuretic, for arthritis, prostatitis, rheumatism, rheumatoid arthritis, high blood pressure and allergic rhinitis.**

The root is recommended as a diuretic, for relief of benign prostatic hyperplasia (BPH) and other prostate problems, and as a natural remedy to treat or prevent baldness.

An infusion of the plant is very valuable in stemming internal bleeding. It is also used to treat anemia, excessive menstruation, hemorrhoids, arthritis, rheumatism and skin complaints, especially eczema. Externally, the plant is used to treat skin complaints, arthritic pain, gout, sciatica, neuralgia, hemorrhoids and hair problems. Taken orally, products made from nettle's aerial parts may interfere with the body's production of prostaglandins and other inflammation-causing chemicals.

Nettle may have an anti-inflammatory effect. It may also enhance responses of the immune system. Chemicals in nettle's aerial parts are also thought to reduce the feeling of pain or interfere with the way that nerves send pain signals. All of these effects may reduce the pain and stiffness of arthritis and other similar conditions.

In addition, Nettle's aerial parts may reduce the amount of histamine that is produced by the body in response to an allergen. An allergen is a substance such as pollen that may provoke an exaggerated immune response in individuals who are sensitive to it. Through this potential action, the aerial parts of Nettle may help to reduce allergy symptoms. Results from one human study are promising, but more research is needed to be conclusive.

A solution of the extract may be applied to the skin to relieve joint pain and muscle aches. Astringent properties of Nettle aerial parts may also help to lessen the swelling of hemorrhoids and stop bleeding from minor skin injuries such as razor nicks. An astringent shrinks and tightens the top layers of skin or mucous membranes, thereby reducing secretions, relieving irritation, and improving tissue firmness. It may also be used topically for dandruff and overly oily hair and scalp. This herb should be used for a minimum of 30 days for full effects.

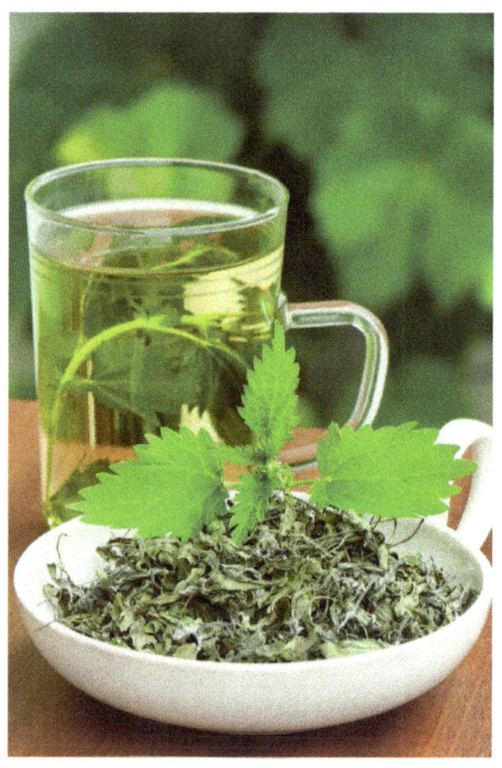

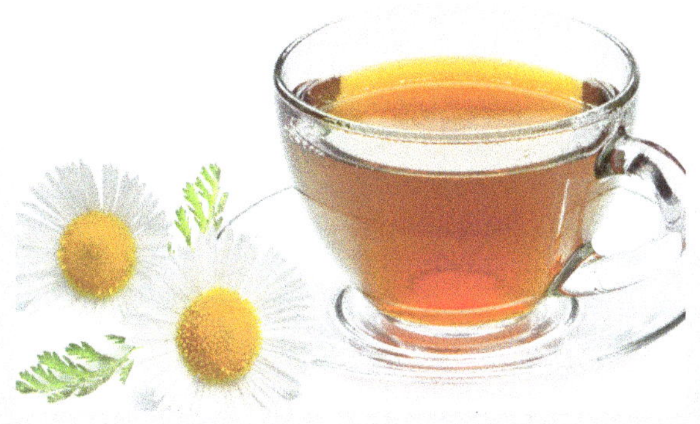

Which Tea is Great for You?

There are so many teas that are good for you in so many ways…there are green teas and Black teas and hundreds of specialty teas. For our purpose, I am sharing some of the basic teas and a list of what is considered to be the top 15 "Home Remedy Teas."

Our Basic Tea

When it comes to herbal, black or green tea, different things suit different people (and a doctor's recommendation should never be overlooked), but for most of us, indulging in a cup or two of black tea might in fact be a healthy life choice, as some studies have shown. Both green and black tea are made from a shrub called Camellia Sinesis, but with different processing methods. In addition to the leaves being withered, rolled and heated, black tea leaves are fermented before the final heating process.

Here are some health benefits of having a cup or two of black tea on a regular basis, though it should be noted that it is recommended that black tea should be consumed without any additives like milk or sugar to truly harness its benefits.

Oral Health:
Studies funded by the Tea Trade Health Research Association, suggests that; black tea reduces plaque formation as well as restricts bacteria growth that promotes the formation of cavities and tooth decays. Polyphenols found in black tea kill and surpass cavity-causing bacteria as well as hinder the growth of bacterial enzymes that form the sticky-like material that binds plaque to our teeth.

A Better Heart:
As identified by Arab L. et al. in their 2009 research paper called "Green and black tea consumption and risk of stroke: a meta-analysis," it is seen that regardless of people's country of origin, individuals who consume 3 or more cups of tea had a 21% lower risk of a stroke than people who consume less than 1 cup of green or black tea per day.

Antioxidants:
Black tea contains polyphenols, which are also antioxidants that help block DNA damage associated with tobacco or other toxic chemicals. These antioxidants are different from those obtained from fruits and vegetables and therefore, as a regular part of our diet, they can provide additional benefits towards a healthy lifestyle.

Cancer Prevention:

Though a lot more research is required to confidently suggest cancer prevention techniques, some research over the years suggests that antioxidants like polyphenol and catechins in tea may help prevent some types of cancer. It has been suggested that women who drink black tea regularly have a lower chance of ovarian cancer than their counterparts.

Healthy Bones:

It has also been suggested that regular tea drinkers have stronger bones and lower probability of developing arthritis due to the phytochemicals found in tea.

Lower Risk of Diabetes:

Based on a research study conducted of elderly people living in the Mediterranean islands; it was discovered that people that had been consuming black tea on a long-term basis on a moderate level (1-2 cups a day) had a 70% lower chance of having or developing Type 2 diabetes.

Stress Relief:

We all are aware, and well experienced, about the calming and relaxing benefits of black tea. Not only does it help slow you down after a long day, studies show that the amino acid L-theanine found in black tea can help you relax and concentrate better. Black tea has also been shown to reduce levels of the stress hormone cortisol when consumed in moderate amounts on a regular basis.

Better Immune System:

Black tea contains alkylamine antigens that help boost our immune response. In addition, it also contains tannins that have the ability to fight viruses and hence, keep us protected from influenza, stomach flu and other such commonly found viruses in our everyday lives.

Healthy Digestive Tract:

In addition to improving your immune system, tannins also have a therapeutic effect on gastric and intestinal illnesses, and also help decrease digestive activity.

Increased Energy:

Unlike other drinks that have relatively higher caffeine content, the low amounts found in tea can help enhance blood flow to the brain without over-stimulating the heart. It also stimulates the metabolism and respiratory system, as well as the heart and the kidneys.

Happiness Factor:

If a perfect cup of tea makes you smile indulge a little, then what could possibly be the harm? As a matter of fact, at least 3 cups of tea a day can boost your inner wellness, so indulge allot.

Sheila Z. Stirling PhD

Why Green Tea?

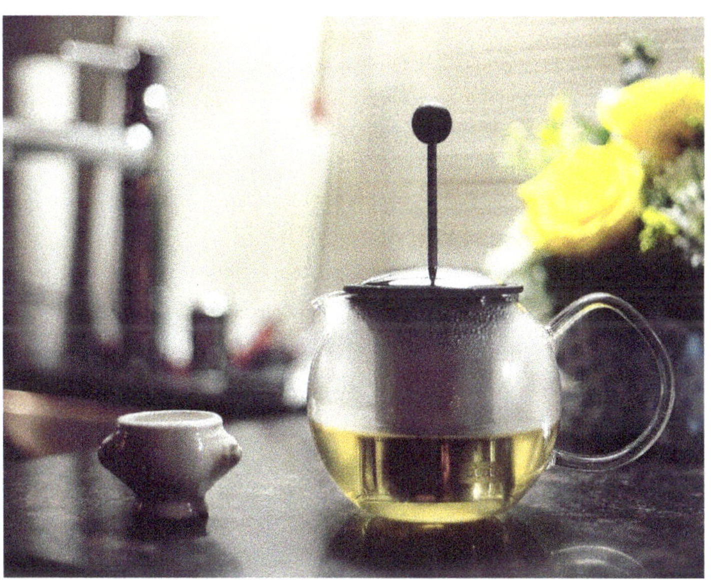

Green tea has been used as a medicine for thousands of years. Originating in China, but widely used throughout Asia, this beverage has a multitude of uses from lowering blood pressure to preventing cancer. The reason that green tea has more health benefits attached to it than black tea, is (apparently) due to the processing. Black tea is processed in a way that allows for fermentation, whereas, green tea's processing avoids the fermentation process.

As a result, green tea retains maximum amount of antioxidants and poly-phenols—the substances that give green tea its many benefits.

Here's a list of some of tea's amazing benefits that you may not have been aware of.

Some of these benefits are still being debated, so please, do your own research if you want to use green tea for medicinal purposes.

- **Weight Loss:** Green tea increases the metabolism. The polyphenol found in green tea works to intensify levels of fat oxidation and the rate at which your body turns food into calories.

- **Diabetes:** Green tea apparently helps regulate glucose levels, slowing the rise of blood sugar after eating. This can prevent high insulin spikes and resulting fat storage.

- **Heart Disease:** Scientists think, green tea works on the lining of blood vessels, helping keep them stay relaxed and better able to withstand changes in blood pressure. It may also protect against the formation of clots, which are the primary cause of heart attacks.

- **Esophageal Cancer:** It can reduce the risk of esophageal cancer, and it is also widely thought to kill cancer cells in general without damaging the healthy tissue around them.

- **Cholesterol:** Green tea reduces bad cholesterol in the blood and improves the ratio of good cholesterol to bad cholesterol.

- **Alzheimer's and Parkinson's:** It is said to delay the deterioration caused by Alzheimer's and

Parkinson's. Studies carried out on mice showed that green tea protected brain cells from dying and restored damaged brain cells.

- Tooth Decay: Studies suggests that the chemical antioxidant "catechin" in tea can destroy bacteria and viruses that cause throat infections, dental caries and other dental conditions.

- Blood Pressure: Regular consumption of green tea is thought to reduce the risk of high blood pressure.

- Depression: Theanine is an amino acid naturally found in tea leaves. It is this substance that is thought to provide a relaxing and tranquilizing effect and be a great benefit to tea drinkers.

- Anti-viral and Anti-bacterial: Tea catechins are strong antibacterial and antiviral agents which make them effective for treating everything from influenza to cancer. In some studies green tea has been shown to inhibit the spread of many diseases.

- Skin care: Green tea can apparently also help with wrinkles and the signs of aging; this is because of its antioxidant and anti-inflammatory activities. Both animal and human studies have demonstrated that green tea applied topically can reduce sun damage.

How Much?

These are some of the many benefits, but the reality is; one cup of tea a day will not give you all the abundant gains. The jury is out on how many cups are necessary; some say as little as two cups a day, while others say five cups—and more still say you can drink up to ten cups a day. If you are thinking of going down this route, you may want to consider taking a green tea supplement instead (it would keep you out of the bathroom).

Another thing to point out is, that there is caffeine in green tea—so if you are sensitive to caffeine, then one cup should be your limit. Green tea also contains tannins (which can decrease the absorption of iron and folic acid), so if you are pregnant or trying to conceive, then green tea may not be ideal for you. You can try mixing green tea with other healthy ingredients such as ginger. For the rest of us—with all these abundant benefits… it's a wonder we drink anything else.
Whether you are lucky enough to grow your own tea herbs, purchase loose teas, or use tea bags, your cabinet is not complete without the following ingredients. These teas are delicious and beneficial, with many different healing qualities. Considering that we most often turn to herbal teas for healing purposes, it's especially important to purchase or grow organic herbs for this purpose. If your leaves are bathed in pesticide and then you add them to boiling water, instead of healing goodness, you are steeping toxins!

When making tea for medicinal purposes, be sure to steep the tea in a teapot with a lid, or to cover your mug while the herbs are steeping. This helps to make a more potent brew by keeping all of the healing oils in the tea, instead of allowing them to drift into the room. Most herbs should be steeped for about 10 minutes for maximum results.

There are many different herbs from around the world that have wonderful healing properties. I've condensed this list to ones that can be easily acquired and stored, or ones that can be easily grown in a backyard garden or a sunny window. Just like band-aids, antibiotic cream, or aspirin, these items are vital additions to your pantry—allowing you to dispense a hot, steaming, fragrant cup of nurturing in as little time as it takes you to boil water. Be prepared by keeping the following ingredients close at hand, and be self-sufficient by producing for yourself, as many as possible. (Growing is always the best way to make sure that they were grown using safe, organic methods.) If you are dealing with a cold or flu, remember how good inhaling the steam from your cup of tea is.

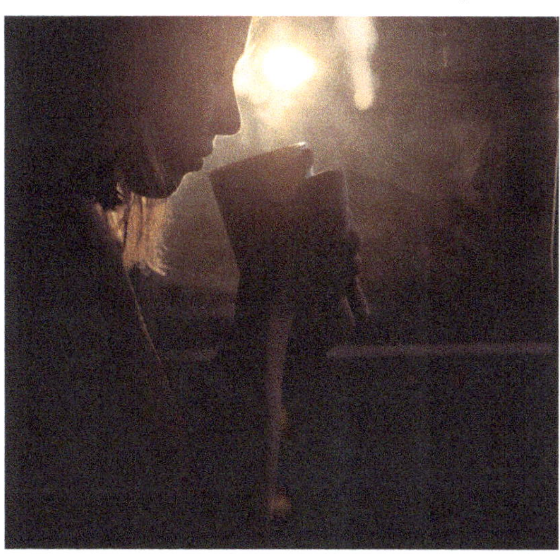

15 Medicinal Teas to Keep on Hand

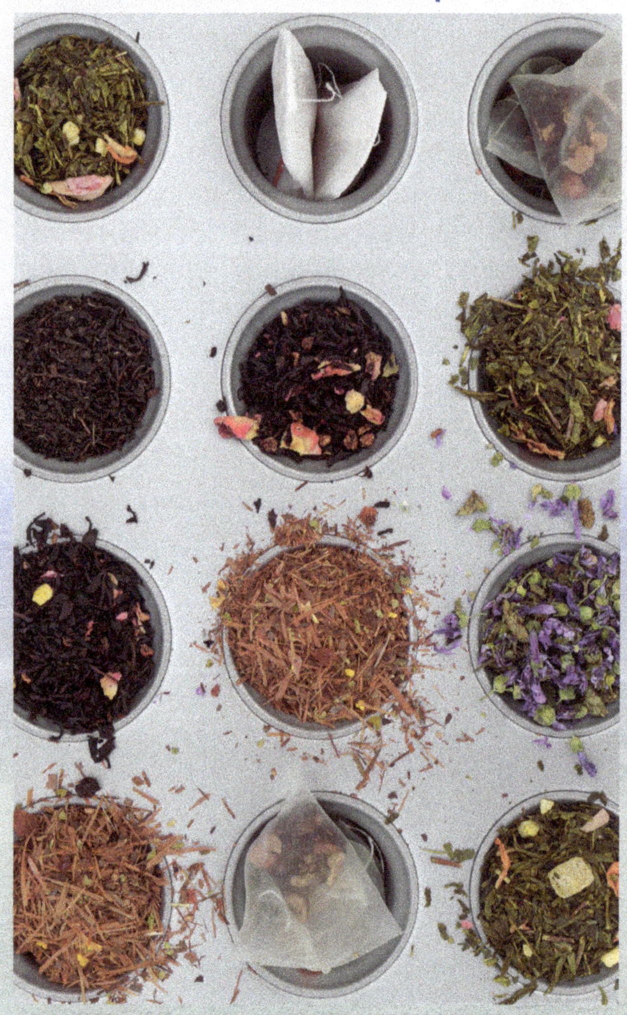

1. Blackberry Leaf

Dried blackberry leaves give a luscious fruity flavor when steeped in boiling water. Not only are they the basis of many delicious teas, they are loaded with a beneficial component called tannins.

Bonus tip: add a blackberry leaf to a jar of pickles when canning—the tannin helps to keep the pickles crisp.

Caution: Excess consumption of blackberry leaves (or anything containing tannins) can cause liver damage.

Blackberry leaf tea can help:

- Provide Vitamin C.

- Treat diarrhea.

- Reduce pain and inflammation from sore throats.

- Provide an antibacterial effect against H-pylori, the bacteria that causes stomach ulcers.

- Provide immune-boosting antioxidants.

- Provide high levels of salicylic acid, which gives them similar properties to aspirin, such as pain relief and fever relief.

- Reduce inflammation of the gums.

2. Chaga Tea

Is a well known cancer fighting mushroom. Chaga tea can be made from 1-2 tsp of Chaga powder in water warmed to 125 degrees. Let it steep for about 10 min. People who drink this tea have reported stronger immune systems, lower cholesterol, better mental clarity and even smoother skin. Chaga is also known for its anti viral properties. This is one powerful mushroom.

3. Chamomile

Chamomile tea should be steeped a little longer than other herbal teas in order to get all of the medicinal benefits. This soothing, slightly apple-flavored tea has mild sedative properties. The petals of the tiny flowers are where the medicinal values lie.

Growing it: Chamomile is easy to grow from seeds. Start them in the late winter and transfer outdoors when the risk of frost has passed. Once the plants are well established, chamomile can thrive with little water during hot weather. When buying your seeds, note that German chamomile is an annual and Roman chamomile is a perennial.

Caution: Chamomile tea should be avoided by people who take blood thinners. As well, those who suffer from ragweed allergies may also have an allergic reaction to chamomile, as the two plants are related.

Chamomile Tea can be used to:
- Relieve anxiety
- Induce sleep
- Soothe mild nausea and indigestion
- Relieve a cough from throat irritation

(Remember not everyone gets along with every herb. I myself do not get along with Chamomile, so I just stay away.)

4. Cinnamon

Cinnamon doesn't just smell like a holiday in a cup, it is anti-bacterial, antiviral, and anti-fungal, making it an excellent all-around remedy for whatever ails you. Cinnamon is a wonderful source of immune-boosting antioxidants.

Growing it: Cinnamon is the fragrant bark of a tropical evergreen tree. This article from Mother Earth Living says; that the trees are surprisingly easy to grow indoors in large pots.

Try this delicious winter beverage:
- 1½ tsp of cinnamon powder or a cinnamon stick
- 1 tea bag
- Honey to taste
- Milk to taste (please use almond milk)

Stir cinnamon powder well into boiling water and steep for 8 minutes. Add a tea bag and steep for 2 more minutes. Stir in honey and warm milk.

Cinnamon Tea can be used to:
- Increase blood flow and improve circulation
- Reduce nausea
- Ease stomach discomfort, bloating, gas and indigestion
- Warm the body from chills
- Soothe a sore throat
- Reduce cold symptoms

5. Clove

Cloves are a wonderful addition to herbal tea just for the taste. Not only is the flavor delicious, but cloves have been used for centuries to treat a variety of ailments. The multipurpose little seed packs a mighty punch with its antiviral, anti-fungal, antimicrobial, antioxidant, and anti-inflammatory properties.

Growing it: Cloves are the dried buds of a flowering evergreen tree that is native to Indonesia, Pakistan, India, Sri Lanka, and Madagascar. They are generally imported and, unfortunately, are not easy to cultivate in other climates or greenhouse atmospheres.

Caution: In high amounts cloves can cause liver damage, blood in the urine, diarrhea, nausea, and dizziness.

Clove tea can help to:
- Provide pain relief–it is a powerful analgesic

- Break up mucous and work as an expectorant

- Provide a fragrant decongestant in a steaming cup of tea

- Treat strep throat or tonsillitis – it relieves pain and provides a wash of antiviral and antibacterial components.

6. Earl Gray
You may be asking why earl grey?
I heard it was just an English tea. The fact is that earl grey contains Bergamot and new studies are showing real promise that bergamot Earl Grey,

is made from black tea and bergamot citrus extract. Compounds in bergamot tea may act as antioxidants, promote healthy digestion, and lower your cholesterol and blood pressure levels. New research is coming out about the main healing aspects of Bergamot.

A word of warning, pure bergamot is strong enough to have an effect on your skin if you put it on your skin. Drinking it with Black tea as to have "Earl Grey" is a safe choice.

7. Echinacea

This lovely flowering plant is probably the pinnacle of herbal preventatives. Echinacea is not only anti-bacterial—but it stimulates the body's immune system to fight off bacterial and viral attacks. The medicinal properties are in the leaves and the purple flowers.

Growing it: Echinacea is also known as the "purple coneflower." The plant has deep taproots and is somewhat drought resistant. It is a perennial. Sow seeds outdoors in the early spring before the last frost. These plants like full sun and they don't like too much moisture.

Echinacea tea can help to:
- Enhance the immune system
- Relieve pain
- Reduce inflammation
- Provide antioxidant effects
- Shorten illness time for the common cold

8. Ginger

This homely root is an ingredient in many natural cough, cold, and nausea treatments. Instead of giving your child ginger-ale when they are suffering from an upset stomach (with all of the high fructose corn syrup and artificial flavors that come in it) brew up a nice cup of ginger tea sweetened with honey for a real dose of soothing ginger!

Growing it: Ginger is a tropical plant that is apparently not difficult to grow indoors. It requires excellent soil, warmth, humidity, and filtered sunlight.

Caution: It's not recommended to exceed 4 grams of ginger per day – components in the herb can cause irritation of the mouth, heartburn and diarrhea if taken in excess. Honey-ginger cough syrup can also be the basis for a nighttime hot toddy.

Ginger tea can be used to:
- Reduce nausea
- Prevent or treat motion sickness
- Warm the body of someone suffering from chills
- Induce sweating to break a fever
- Soothe a sore throat

9. Hawthorne Berry Tea

Hawthorn is a flowering shrub or tree of the rose family. Historically, hawthorn has been used for heart disease as well as for digestive and kidney problems. It has also been used for anxiety.

Here are 9 impressive health benefits of hawthorn berry.

- Loaded with antioxidants.
- May have anti-inflammatory properties.
- May lower blood pressure.
- May decrease blood fats.
- Used to aid digestion.
- Helps prevent hair loss.
- May reduce anxiety.
- Used to treat heart failure.
- Many feel it strengthens the heart muscle.

10. Hibiscus Tea

Hibiscus is actually a flower that is dried and made into a tea. Historically, hibiscus tea has been used in African countries to decrease body temperature, treat heart disease, and sooth a sore throat. Recent studies have looked at the possible role of hibiscus in the treatment of high blood pressure and high cholesterol.

Packed With Antioxidants Hibiscus may Help:
- Lower Blood Pressure
- Lower Blood Fat Levels
- Boost Liver Health
- Promote Weight Loss
- Help Prevent Cancer
- Help Fight Bacteria

11. Lemon Balm

Lemon balm, also known as Bee Balm, was first recorded to have been used by the ancient Greeks as an overall tonic for good health. It is an ingredient in the old world Carmelite water, a recipe created by Carmelite nuns in the early 1600's to treat headaches. (The traditional mixture also contained coriander, lemon-peel, nutmeg, and angelica root.)

Growing it: Lemon balm is easy to grow and produces throughout the summer. The more you harvest, the more it produces. It is perennial in warmer climates. Lemon balm likes rich moist soil with organic compost and partial shade in the hottest part of the day. It is another one of those herbs that can take over a garden, so plant it in a confined area.

Lemon balm tea can help to:
- Fight off viruses – it was used historically against shingles, mumps, and cold sores
- Calm anxiety and nervousness
- Aid in sleep
- Aid the digestive system by reducing spasms and quelling heartburn
- Reduce nausea

12. Lemongrass

Lemongrass is another herb that is loaded with healing properties. The spiky, easy to grow plant has antibacterial, anti-inflammatory, anti-parasitic, and anti-fungal properties, making it helpful in treating a plethora of ailments.

Growing it: You can actually root the lemongrass that you buy at the grocery store to start your own patio lemongrass farm. It grows beautifully in a large pot, making it a good herb for the apartment windowsill farmer to cultivate. It can be grown year round indoors.

Lemongrass Tea can help to:
- Aid in digestion

- Calm nervous disorders and anxiety
- Aid in the treatment of high blood pressure if a daily cup is enjoyed
- Dilate blood vessels and improve circulation
- Act as a mild diuretic to reduce fluid retention

13. Mint or Peppermint

Mint tea is the classic herbal tea. Mint is an ingredient in many different commercial tea blends and is much loved for its refreshing fragrance.

Growing it: Mint is an herb that doesn't just grow easily—it can quickly overtake your garden! For this reason, it is recommended to grow mint in either a container or its own bed. There are many varieties of mint, and the healing properties are similar. Whether you grow peppermint or spearmint, the active component is menthol.

Caution: If you suffer from acid reflux, mint tea may worsen your symptoms. Mint has antispasmodic properties.

Mint tea can be used to:
- Reduce congestion in a cold or flu sufferer
- Reduce pain and bloating from gas
- Reduce cramping from diarrhea
- Act as a mild expectorant for a chest cold or bronchitis Induce sweating, the body's natural cooling mechanism. This is a natural way to reduce a fever
- Relieve nausea without vomiting

14. Pine Needle Tea

Did you know Pine Needle tea was used by indigenous people in North America upwards of a thousand yeas ago. The best benefits of pine needle tea include maximizing the immune system, improving vision, preventing respiratory infections, stimulating circulation.

Caution: As pine needles are not safe to eat or drink. Look for pine needles that grow in clusters of 5 or buy it already packaged as tea. Great for healing from bronchial infections. A high vitamin C and vitamin A content along with various B vitamins makes this a great recovery tea.

15. Rosehips

Rosehips make a tart, tangy pink-colored tea. They are the seed-filled pod at the base of a rose blossom, giving you a practical reason to have more rose bushes in your garden. It mixes well and enhances the flavor of any berry or fruit-flavored tea.

Rosehip tea can help to:
* Provide a nutritional supplement of Vitamin C
* Improve adrenal function
* Boost the immune system
* Provide minerals such as calcium, iron, silicon, selenium, natural sodium, magnesium, manganese, potassium, phosphorus and zinc
* Increase energy

In Closing

There are a few things to remember.
1. You are the captain of your own ship.

2. Every choice you make can move you closer to a vibrant and healthy life or move you in the opposite direction, from illness and death.

3. Rome wasn't built in a day, however I will share with you that 100% of the people that actually do and complete my 8 weeks to wellness program experience major changes for the better in all aspects in their life. From illness to wellness in just 8 weeks.

This writing is meant to inspire you and share with you many tips and truthful information that can assist in bringing you to a healthier and more balanced way of thinking about food and herbs and teas.

Yes, food can be medicine if it is clean food. So seek the highest quality and reach for the stars because you are an amazing human and only you can change the form you are standing in.

With love and blessings,
Sheila Z

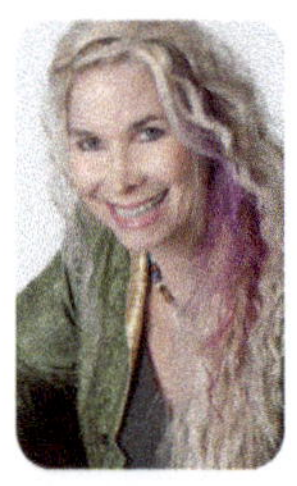

About the Author

Sheila Z is more than an award winning author, amazing whole food chef and creator of *"True Life Solutions" and "8 weeks to Wellness"* and many other programs. Sheila is dedicated to helping people live healthier lives. Her connection to mother nature and her respect for the land and all living things is unique and filled with wisdom beyond her years. Sheila has helped countless people worldwide gain a deeper understanding to the causes of their life challenges.

Sheila Z is . . .

- A PhD in Natural Health/Philosophy
- Creator of *True Life Solutions* & Vibrant Life Cook Book and The 8 Weeks to Wellness Program
- Developed the Vibrant Life Protocol™
  "The Intentional Wellness Experience™"
- Certified Nutritional Live Blood Microscopist
- An International Inspirational Speaker & Catalyst for Youngevity
- Reiki Master
- An Emotional Clarity Specialist
- Energy Specialist
- Certified Lymphologist
- Ordained Minister
- Master Meditation Instructor
- Intuitive
- Certified Light & Sound Healer
- Acutonics Practitioner

Through years of study and working with clients, Sheila has become an expert in emotional clarity and is a catalyst for healing and wellness. She is a Spiritual Evolutionist, and has an on-going practice in Las Vegas, Nevada. Sheila is a Healing, Wellness, and Relationship coach. Her meditations have helped countless people find their gifts and their purpose. She has enriched the lives of many with her insights and grace.

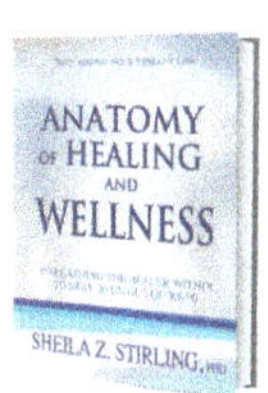

Anatomy of Healing and Wellness

268 full color pages of ways to improve your Health and Wellness. An in depth guide, resource and cutting edge information on how to stay 30 till you are 90! From Physical form of Wellness to the Science of Wellness and the Emotional aspect of Wellness. Using foods as medicine and so much more.

"This book is amazing as it shows you what herbs, teas and natural sources can help to heal whatever ails you. A great book on preventing illness and on recovery."

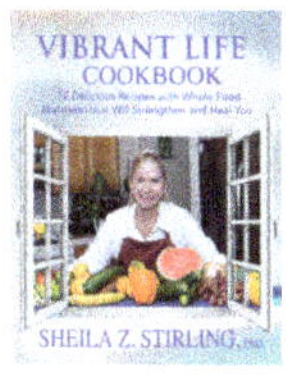

Vibrant Life Cookbook

Can you change your health in 100 days? YES! Vastly improve the conditions of your blood and get your body back into balance. This program is not for the faint of heart. If you want to avoid illness, want to strengthen your system and stay "30 til you are 90" this is the program for you. An in-depth discovery session is required before starting this protocol. Each protocol is explicitly for one person. You! Contact Dr. Stirling for an apt.

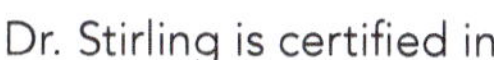

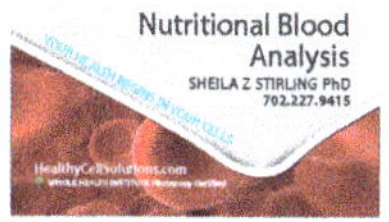

Dr. Stirling is certified in
"Nutritional Live Blood Microscopy"
You can email her for an appointment:

info@HealthyCellSolutions.com

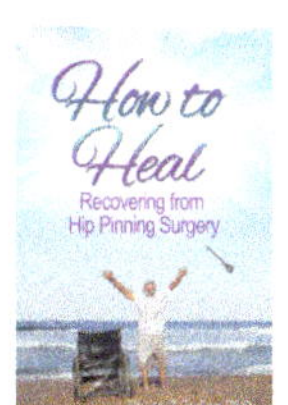

Recovering from Hip Pinning Surgery

This amazing full color booklet gives you important information and a step-by-step guide on how to best recover from major surgery like hip pinning. A useful guide and inspiration for those going into a surgical procedure.

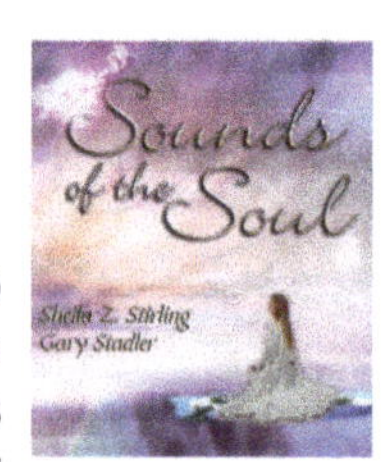

Sounds of the Soul CD

When listened through headphones, this CD seems to balance Alpha, Beta, Theta, and Delta brainwaves. The implications of this are boundless and as we know that meditation has the ability to decrease blood pressure and stress levels. We now know that Sounds of the Soul may potentially normalize brain function and, in doing so, heal the body on a cellular and soulular level. The sounds and tones are very relaxing and channel directly to the soul, so open your heart and breathe in the music. Many have experienced a reconnection with spirit and accelerated healing.
Go to www.SoundsoftheSoul.com
or contact Sheila Z

Cutting edge scientific studies are now being done with neuro-feedback EEGs and the initial findings are astounding. Sounds of the Soul was channeled from the celestial realm through Sheila Z. It is an interpretation of the God code of creation in collaboration with Gary Stadler of HeartMagic Studios. There are 2 tracks on this CD one is 18:50 minutes and the other is 27:24 minutes.

Deep Healing Meditation with The Sounds of the Soul CD

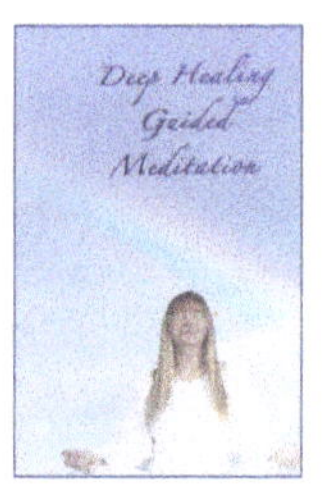

This is a journey meditation that encourages your connection to the healer within. Building the healing energy of the cosmos and being in the heightened vibrations of the angelic realms from *Sounds of the Soul.* This meditation is about 27 minutes.
Email Sheila Z - Sheilaz@truelife-solutions.com

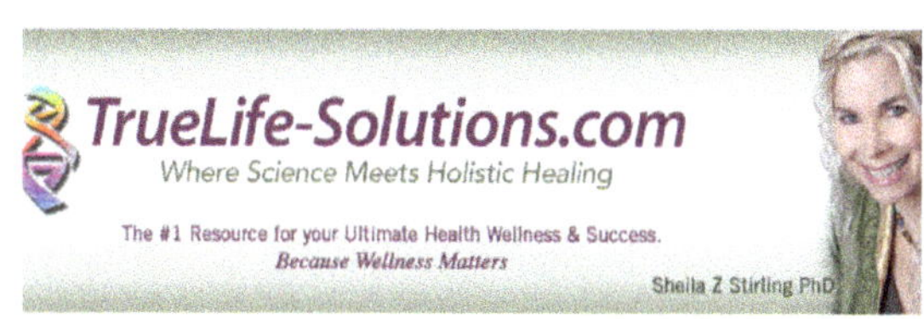

Sheila Z Stirling is dedicated to healing the planet and raising the consciousness of humanity. This has been a diverse journey, from Ancient ways to Quantum Physics, from Philosophy to Alchemy. Below are web sites created by Sheila Z Stirling for the advancement, education and accelerated healing for all. Sheila is an Environmental Activist and has lobbied for the national parks in Washington D.C. Sheila is the Southern Nevada coordinator for the Institute of Noetic Sciences - Bridging Science and Consciousness.

Sheila Z's sites:

TrueLife-Solutions.com - Sheila Z's main web site on health and wellness.
TrueEMFSolutions.com - This site is dedicated to protection from EMF's.
HealthyCellSolutions.com - This site has the tried and true health products that are the favorites of True Life-Solutions and Sheila Z.
YosemiteEbook.com - A beautiful book about Yosemite, photos and writings by Sheila Z.
LoveandIllusion.com - This award winning book written by Dr. Stirling covers the subject of sociopathic behavior in relationships.
IONSLasVegas.com - The site for the community group "Bridging Science and Consciousness."
ZenGems.net - Healing Stone Jewelry designed and created by Sheila Z.
Whatsupwithplanetearth.org - Information on Mother Earth.
AnatomyofHealingandWellness.com - The website for Sheila Z's amazing holistic health resource book.
Pro-Tec-Ted.com - EMF & Wave Protection
SavingWildHorsesNevada.com

" Sheila Z Stirling is a wonderful presenter, inspirational motivational speaker. Her knowledge of the human form and the path to regain complete wellness has helped achieve great success for so many. Please contact Sheila for more information on having her speak at your group, company gathering. Consider booking an in-depth Discovery session. I understand it can be life changing for the better. I have known Dr. Stirling for many years and have experienced and benefited from her knowledge, her wisdom and her teachings."
— Dr. Stephen Ezra West, DL - www.zerodisease.com

An Ounce of Prevention

Discovering

The How...The Why & The What of

Prevention

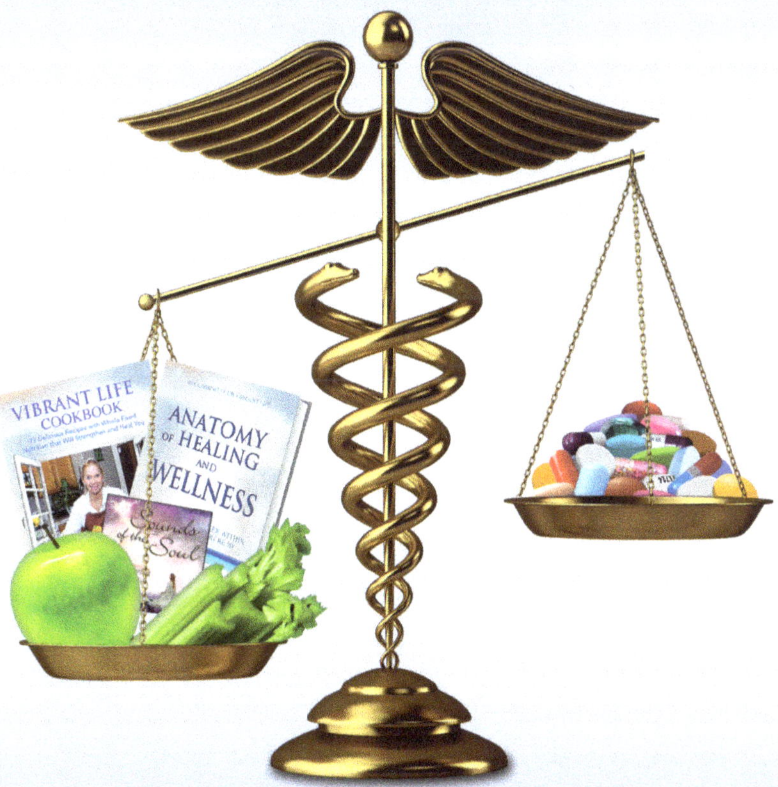

Sheila Z Stirling PhD

An Ounce of Prevention
by Sheila Z. Stirling PhD
Copyright ©2020

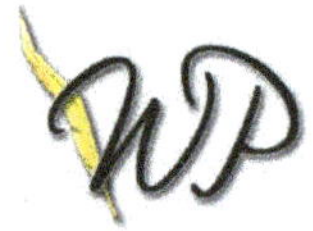

Wisdom Press Publishing
4132 S. Rainbow Blvd. #465
Las Vegas, NV 89103
www.wisdompresspublishing.com

Sheila Z. Stirling, PhD
ISBN 9780991102679

Library of Congress: 2020

Printed in the United States of America

Cover Design by Thayer D.
Sheila Z and Jonathon
Interior layout by Dianne Leonetti-Rux - DzinerGraphics.com